Advances in Diagnosis and Therapy of Neuroendocrine Neoplasms

Advances in Diagnosis and Therapy of Neuroendocrine Neoplasms

Editor

Eva Segelov

MDPI • Basel • Beijing • Wuhan • Barcelona • Belgrade • Manchester • Tokyo • Cluj • Tianjin

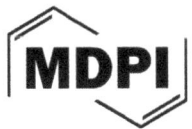

Editor
Eva Segelov
Monash Health and Monash University
Australia

Editorial Office
MDPI
St. Alban-Anlage 66
4052 Basel, Switzerland

This is a reprint of articles from the Special Issue published online in the open access journal *Journal of Clinical Medicine* (ISSN 2077-0383) (available at: https://www.mdpi.com/journal/jcm/special_issues/Neuroendocrine_Neoplasms).

For citation purposes, cite each article independently as indicated on the article page online and as indicated below:

LastName, A.A.; LastName, B.B.; LastName, C.C. Article Title. *Journal Name* **Year**, *Volume Number*, Page Range.

ISBN 978-3-03943-745-0 (Hbk)
ISBN 978-3-03943-746-7 (PDF)

© 2020 by the authors. Articles in this book are Open Access and distributed under the Creative Commons Attribution (CC BY) license, which allows users to download, copy and build upon published articles, as long as the author and publisher are properly credited, which ensures maximum dissemination and a wider impact of our publications.

The book as a whole is distributed by MDPI under the terms and conditions of the Creative Commons license CC BY-NC-ND.

Contents

About the Editor vii

Preface to "Advances in Diagnosis and Therapy of Neuroendocrine Neoplasms" ix

Valentina Andreasi, Stefano Partelli, Gabriele Capurso, Francesca Muffatti, Gianpaolo Balzano, Stefano Crippa and Massimo Falconi
Long-Term Pancreatic Functional Impairment after Surgery for Neuroendocrine Neoplasms
Reprinted from: *J. Clin. Med.* 2019, 8, 1611, doi:10.3390/jcm8101611 1

Braden Woodhouse, Sharon Pattison, Eva Segelov, Simron Singh, Kate Parker, Grace Kong, William Macdonald, David Wyld, Goswin Meyer-Rochow, Nick Pavlakis, Siobhan Conroy, Vallerie Gordon, Jonathan Koea, Nicole Kramer, Michael Michael, Kate Wakelin, Tehmina Asif, Dorothy Lo, Timothy Price, Ben Lawrence and on behalf of the Commonwealth Neuroendocrine Tumour Collaboration (CommNETs)
Consensus-Derived Quality Performance Indicators for Neuroendocrine Tumour Care
Reprinted from: *J. Clin. Med.* 2019, 8, 1455, doi:10.3390/jcm8091455 15

Salvatore Tafuto, Claudia von Arx, Monica Capozzi, Fabiana Tatangelo, Manuela Mura, Roberta Modica, Maria Luisa Barretta, Antonella Di Sarno, Maria Lina Tornesello, Annamaria Colao and Alessandro Ottaiano
Safety and Activity of Metronomic Temozolomide in Second-Line Treatment of Advanced Neuroendocrine Neoplasms
Reprinted from: *J. Clin. Med.* 2019, 8, 1224, doi:10.3390/jcm8081224 - 27

Ludovica Magi, Federica Mazzuca, Maria Rinzivillo, Giulia Arrivi, Emanuela Pilozzi, Daniela Prosperi, Elsa Iannicelli, Paolo Mercantini, Michele Rossi, Patrizia Pizzichini, Andrea Laghi, Alberto Signore, Paolo Marchetti, Bruno Annibale and Francesco Panzuto
Multidisciplinary Management of Neuroendocrine Neoplasia: A Real-World Experience from a Referral Center
Reprinted from: *J. Clin. Med.* 2019, 8, 910, doi:10.3390/jcm8060910 37

Deise Uema, Carolina Alves, Marcella Mesquita, Jose Eduardo Nuñez, Timo Siepmann, Martin Angel, Juliana F. M. Rego, Rui Weschenfelder, Duilio R. Rocha Filho, Frederico P. Costa, Milton Barros, Juan M. O'Connor, Ben M. Illigens and Rachel P. Riechelmann
Carcinoid Heart Disease and Decreased Overall Survival among Patients with Neuroendocrine Tumors: A Retrospective Multicenter Latin American Cohort Study
Reprinted from: *J. Clin. Med.* 2019, 8, 405, doi:10.3390/jcm8030405 45

Enes Kaçmaz, Charlotte M. Heidsma, Marc G. H. Besselink, Koen M. A. Dreijerink, Heinz-Josef Klümpen, Elisabeth J. M. Nieveen van Dijkum and Anton F. Engelsman
Treatment of Liver Metastases from Midgut Neuroendocrine Tumours: A Systematic Review and Meta-Analysis
Reprinted from: *J. Clin. Med.* 2019, 8, 403, doi:10.3390/jcm8030403 57

Melissa Frizziero, Bipasha Chakrabarty, Bence Nagy, Angela Lamarca, Richard A. Hubner, Juan W. Valle and Mairéad G. McNamara
Mixed Neuroendocrine Non-Neuroendocrine Neoplasms: A Systematic Review of a Controversial and Underestimated Diagnosis
Reprinted from: *J. Clin. Med.* 2020, 9, 273, doi:10.3390/jcm9010273 71

.Angela Lamarca, Hamish Clouston, Jorge Barriuso, Mairéad G McNamara,
Melissa Frizziero, Was Mansoor, Richard A Hubner, Prakash Manoharan, Sarah O'Dwyer
and Juan W Valle
Follow-Up Recommendations after Curative Resection of Well-Differentiated Neuroendocrine
Tumours: Review of Current Evidence and Clinical Practice
Reprinted from: *J. Clin. Med.* **2019**, *8*, 1630, doi:10.3390/jcm8101630 . . . . **95**

Claudia von Arx, Monica Capozzi, Elena López-Jiménez, Alessandro Ottaiano,
Fabiana Tatangelo, Annabella Di Mauro, Guglielmo Nasti, Maria Lina Tornesello and
Salvatore Tafuto
Updates on the Role of Molecular Alterations and NOTCH Signalling in the Development of
Neuroendocrine Neoplasms
Reprinted from: *J. Clin. Med.* **2019**, *8*, 1277, doi:10.3390/jcm8091277 . . . . **111**

About the Editor

Eva Segelov was appointed as Professor and Director of Oncology at Monash Health and Monash University in February 2017. She is an Honorary Associate of the NHMRC Clinical Trials Centre, Sydney Medical School, and Honorary Professor at Shanghai Jiao Tong University; she was previously Associate Professor at the University of New South Wales and Senior Medical Oncologist at St Vincent's Hospital, Sydney. She is a recognised national and international expert in the fields of gastrointestinal cancer, including neuroendocrine tumours and breast cancer, with a 20 year history of patient management in a multidisciplinary setting. Professor Segelov is an active member of the Australian Gastrointestinal Trials Group (AGITG), and served as a Board Member and Convenor of the Annual Scientific Meeting 2014–2018. She is the co-founder of the Commonwealth Neuroendocrine Tumour Society (CommNETS), an international research collaborative; Chair of the Gastrointestinal Group of the Clinical Oncological Society of Australia (COSA); faculty group member of the European Society of Medical Oncology (ESMO) CUP, Endocrine Tumours, and Others group and the Gastrointestinal Faculty Group; IDMSC member for Trans-Tasman Oncology Group (TROG). She is an Associate Editor of the Journal of Global Oncology (ASCO) and Guest Editor of its Inaugural Special Edition, "Cancer in Indigenous Communities". Eva serves on the ESMO Annual Scientific Meeting subcommittee Neuroendocrine and Endocrine cancer and is a member of the conference organizing committee for the inaugural ASCO "Breakthrough: A Global Summit for Oncology Innovators meeting" conference; she was co-Track Chair of Gastrointestinal Cancer for the 2017 ESMO Asia Annual Scientific Meeting.

Preface to "Advances in Diagnosis and Therapy of Neuroendocrine Neoplasms"

This Special Issue is dedicated to neuroendocrine neoplasms (NENs), a category of malignancy that demonstrates wide clinical heterogeneity, posing major challenges in diagnosis and management. There have been significant advances in the field of NEN genomics, pathology, imaging, and treatment over the past five years. NENs are examples of rare tumours (although their incidence and prevalence are increasing) where international collaborative efforts have allowed the generation of high-level evidence to guide optimal patient-centred care. This issue presents both reviews and original papers to provide comprehensive state-of-the-art understanding of this fascinating disease.

Eva Segelov
Editor

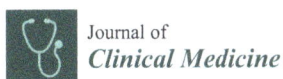

Article

Long-Term Pancreatic Functional Impairment after Surgery for Neuroendocrine Neoplasms

Valentina Andreasi [1,2,†], Stefano Partelli [1,2,†], Gabriele Capurso [3], Francesca Muffatti [1], Gianpaolo Balzano [1], Stefano Crippa [1,2] and Massimo Falconi [1,2,*]

[1] Pancreatic Surgery Unit, Pancreas Translational & Clinical Research Center, San Raffaele Scientific Institute IRCCS, 20132 Milan, Italy; andreasi.valentina@hsr.it (V.A.); partelli.stefano@hsr.it (S.P.); muffatti.francesca@hsr.it (F.M.); balzano.gianpaolo@hsr.it (G.B.); crippa1.stefano@hsr.it (S.C.)
[2] Faculty of Medicine and Surgery, "Vita-Salute San Raffaele" University, 20132 Milan, Italy
[3] Biliopancreatic Endoscopy Unit, Pancreas Translational & Clinical Research Center, San Raffaele Scientific Institute IRCCS, 20132 Milan, Italy; capurso.gabriele@hsr.it
* Correspondence: falconi.massimo@hsr.it; Tel.: +39-02-2643-6020
† Valentina Andreasi and Stefano Partelli share the first authorship.

Received: 30 August 2019; Accepted: 27 September 2019; Published: 3 October 2019

Abstract: Radical surgery represents the only curative treatment for pancreatic neuroendocrine neoplasms (PanNEN). The aim of this study was to evaluate the postoperative onset of diabetes mellitus (DM) and/or pancreatic exocrine insufficiency (PEI) in surgically treated PanNEN. Consecutive PanNEN patients, without preoperative DM, who underwent partial pancreatic resection, were included. After a median follow-up of 72 months, overall 68/276 patients (24%) developed DM. Patients who developed DM were significantly older ($p = 0.002$) and they had a higher body mass index (BMI) ($p < 0.0001$) than those who did not; they were more frequently male ($p = 0.017$) and with nonfunctioning neoplasms ($p = 0.019$). BMI > 25 Kg/m^2 was the only independent predictor of DM ($p = 0.001$). Overall, 118/276 patients (43%) developed a PEI, which was significantly more frequent after pancreaticoduodenectomy ($p < 0.0001$) and in patients with T3-T4 tumors ($p = 0.001$). Pancreaticoduodenectomy was the only independent predictor of PEI ($p < 0.0001$). Overall, 54 patients (20%) developed disease progression. Patients with and without DM had similar progression free survival (PFS), whereas patients without PEI had better five-year-PFS ($p = 0.002$), although this association was not confirmed in multivariate analysis. The risk of DM and PEI after surgery for PanNEN is relatively high but it does not affect PFS. BMI and pancreatic head resection are independent predictors of DM and PEI, respectively.

Keywords: pancreatic neuroendocrine neoplasms; neuroendocrine tumor; long-term functional outcomes; pancreatectomy; diabetes mellitus; pancreatic exocrine insufficiency; body mass index; parenchyma-sparing surgery

1. Introduction

Pancreatic neuroendocrine neoplasms (PanNEN) represent less than 3% of all pancreatic lesions. Despite being still considered rare tumors, their incidence has dramatically increased during the last two decades, which is probably due to the widespread use of high-quality imaging techniques [1,2]. PanNEN exhibit heterogeneous biological behaviour, which ranges from indolent to aggressive forms. Overall, the survival rates for PanNEN are better than those that were reported for their exocrine counterpart. The vast majority of PanNEN is represented by well-differentiated forms (PanNET) with a reported five-year survival rate of 70–90% for patients with localized PanNEN that decreases to 40–60% for patients with metastatic disease [3–5]. Radical surgery represents the backbone for the curative treatment of PanNEN [6]. Therefore, given the good prognosis and the high rate of cure of these neoplasms, it is of paramount importance to carefully weigh the oncological risk along with the long-term functional outcomes following pancreatic resection. In particular, the onset of diabetes mellitus (DM) and/or pancreatic exocrine insufficiency (PEI) might have a considerable impact on the general health status and on the quality of life of these patients [7,8]. At this regard, it has been reported that malnutrition that results from PEI can lead to the development of comorbidities that negatively impact on prognosis [9,10]. For these reasons, parenchyma-sparing surgical procedures (i.e., enucleation and middle pancreatectomy) have been proposed for reducing the incidence of postoperative pancreatic endocrine and exocrine insufficiency [11–14] and it has been widely reported that parenchyma-sparing surgery, enucleation in particular [15,16], is associated to improved long-term functional outcomes as compared to formal resections [11,16–19]. The likelihood of developing pancreatic insufficiency depends on the extent of pancreatic resection as well as on the functionality of the remaining parenchyma [19]. Several studies, investigating patients with different benign or low-grade malignant lesions, have shown that the type of surgical procedure (parenchyma-sparing vs. standard resection), but also other patients' related factors, such as age or the presence of chronic pancreatitis, might contribute to the post-surgical development of pancreatic insufficiency [19–21].

Aim of the present study was to evaluate the rate of long-term pancreatic impairment, defined as postoperative onset of DM and/or of PEI, in a series of patients submitted to partial pancreatic resection for PanNEN and investigate factors that are associated with it. The secondary aim was to evaluate a possible effect of pancreatic insufficiency on progression free survival (PFS).

2. Experimental Section

2.1. Study Design

This retrospective cohort study was conducted following the Strengthening the Reporting of Observational Studies in Epidemiology Statement (STROBE) guidelines [22]. All of the patients who underwent surgery for PanNEN at San Raffaele Scientific Institute (Milan) between January 2002 and December 2017 were retrospectively screened. Patients submitted to partial pancreatic resection (pancreaticoduodenectomy (PD), distal pancreatectomy (DP), atypical resection (AR)) for PanNEN with available long-term functional outcomes data were included in the study. Patients with a preoperative diagnosis of DM and/or PEI as well as those who underwent total pancreatectomy for PanNEN, were excluded from the present study. Patients submitted to enucleation were also excluded, as this surgical procedure, which consisted in the removal of just the tumor without resecting pancreatic parenchyma, could not be considered as a partial pancreatic resection. Patients who deceased within 90 days from operation due to surgical complications were also excluded. Figure 1 depicts the initial number of patients who were screened and the final study population.

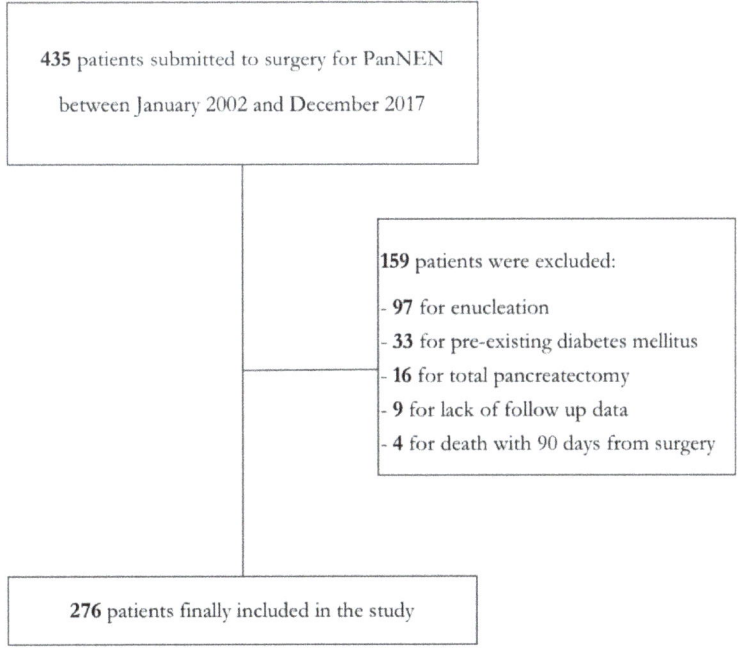

Figure 1. Flowchart representing patients included in the study.

2.2. Definition of Outcomes

The postoperative onset of DM and PEI represented the main outcome of this study. According to the American Diabetes Association diagnostic criteria [23], postoperative DM was defined when glycated haemoglobin (HbA1c) was equal to or greater than 6.5% and/or in the presence of a fasting plasma glucose (FPG) equal to or greater than 126 mg/dL and/or in a patient with classic symptoms of hyperglycemia or hyperglycemic crisis associated to a random plasma glucose that was equal to or greater than 200 mg/dL. FPG and HbA1c were measured in all of the patients before surgery. PEI was diagnosed in the presence of manifest clinical signs of malabsorption and/or maldigestion (steatorrhea, weight loss, flatulence, and abdominal distention), which improved with the assumption of pancreatic enzyme replacement therapy. The secondary outcome of this study was represented by the possible effect of pancreatic insufficiency on PFS.

All of the patients were followed up regularly after surgery. High-quality imaging examination, as well as blood tests inclusive of HbA1c and FPG, were performed at least every six months (in the absence of signs or symptoms of hyperglycemia). A follow-up phone call was scheduled on a six-month basis, whereas an outpatient visit was planned on a yearly basis. Information regarding general health status and possible signs or symptoms of pancreatic insufficiency was collected during outpatient visits or by telephone. Last follow up was updated in June 2019. Progression free survival (PFS) was defined as the time from surgery to the first evidence of disease recurrence or progression and it was censored at the last follow up if no disease relapse had occurred. Overall survival (OS) was defined as the time from surgery to death and censored at the last follow up if no events had happened.

2.3. Data Collection

Demographic data, perioperative details, and pathological findings were retrospectively retrieved from an electronic database. Preoperative variables considered were: age, gender, body mass index (BMI), tumor functionality, and the presence of an inherited syndrome. The choice of the surgical technique was based on the location, the size, and the preoperative aggressiveness features of the neoplasm. PD and DP were routinely performed for tumors that were located in the head and in the body-tail of the pancreas, respectively. Middle pancreatectomy was performed in the presence of small tumors < 4 cm, which could not be removed by enucleation, located in the pancreatic neck/proximal body and without features of aggressiveness. Middle-preserving pancreatectomy was chosen in the presence of a multifocal disease (i.e., multiple endocrine neoplasia (MEN) type 1) involving pancreatic head and tail, but skipping the body of the gland [24]. Islet autotransplantation was carried out, although not routinely, in patients requiring a DP for a benign/borderline PanNEN located in the pancreatic body/neck [25]. This procedure started being performed in January 2009 and it is still ongoing. The Clavien-Dindo classification system was used to assess the severity of postoperative complications [26]. The rates of postoperative pancreatic fistula (POPF) [27], abdominal collection, hemoperitoneum, blood transfusion, and readmission were evaluated. Length of hospital stay (LOS) and operative time were also considered. At final histology, PanNEN were classified according to the current TNM European NeuroEndocrine Tumor Society (ENETS) classification [28]. Ki67 proliferative index was assessed in the surgical specimen by MIB1 antibody staining and evaluated by measuring the percentage of cells with positive nuclear staining after the count of 2000 cells in the area of highest nuclear labelling [3]. Tumor grade was defined according to the 2017 World Health organization (WHO) Classification [3].

2.4. Statistical Analysis

Continuous variables were expressed as mean and standard deviation (SD) for normally distributed data and as median and interquartile range (IQR) for skewed distributions. The categorical variables were presented as numbers and percentages (%). The comparison between subgroups was performed using Student's *t* test or Mann-Whitney U test, for continuous variables as appropriate. Qualitative data were compared by the Chi square test or Fisher's exact test, when appropriate. Multivariate logistic regression analysis was performed to evaluate the predictors of postoperative DM and of PEI. Survival probability was estimated according to the Kaplan-Meier method. Multivariate analysis to evaluate significant predictors of PFS was performed by the Cox regression model. Follow-up was updated on June 2019, giving a potential minimum follow-up of 18 months to each patient. Statistical analyses were performed in SPSS 25.0 for Mac (SPSS Inc., Chicago, IL, USA). p values were considered to be significant when less or equal than 0.05.

3. Results

3.1. Study Population

Overall, 276 patients were included in the present study. Of these, 76 patients (27%) underwent PD, whereas 192 (70%) were submitted to DP. Atypical parenchyma-sparing resections were performed in the remaining eight cases (3%) ($n = 7$ middle pancreatectomy, $n = 1$ middle-preserving pancreatectomy). Table 1 summarizes perioperative details.

Table 1. Perioperative details of 276 patients submitted to surgery for pancreatic neuroendocrine neoplasms (PanNEN).

Variable	n (%)
Operative time, min [1]	240 (180;300)
Length of stay, days [1]	9 (7;11)
Readmission	
No	242 (88)
Yes	34 (12)

Table 1. Cont.

Variable	n (%)
Blood transfusion	
No	229 (83)
Yes	47 (17)
Islet autotransplatation	
No	267 (97)
Yes	9 (3)
Complications [26]	
No complications	94 (34)
I	56 (20)
II	89 (32)
III	36 (13)
IV	1 (1)
POPF [27]	
No	147 (53)
Yes	129 (47)
Abdominal Collection	
No	223 (81)
Yes	53 (19)
Postoperative Hemorrhage	
No	262 (95)
Yes	14 (5)

[1] Expressed as median [interquartile range (IQR)]. POPF: Postoperative Pancreatic Fistula.

3.2. Postoperative DM

At a median follow-up of 72 months (IQR 38;103 months) after surgery, 68 patients (24%) developed a postoperative DM. Table 2 reports a comparison of demographic, perioperative and pathological characteristics between patients who developed DM and those who did not. Patients who developed DM were significantly older when compared to those who did not develop DM (median 60 years (IQR 56;67 years) vs. 56 years (IQR 46;67 years), $p = 0.002$). The median preoperative BMI was significantly higher in patients who developed postoperative diabetes (median 27 Kg/m^2 (25;30 Kg/m^2) vs. 24 Kg/m^2 (IQR 22;27 Kg/m^2), $p < 0.0001$). Postoperative DM presented more frequently in males than in females ($p = 0.017$), as well as in patients that were diagnosed with nonfunctioning neoplasms as compared to patients with functioning tumors ($p = 0.019$). In the group of patients who developed DM, functioning PanNEN ($n = 6$) were insulinomas in five cases (83%) and a VIPoma in one case. The rate of postoperative diabetes was similar between patients submitted to different surgical procedures ($p = 0.476$). Among those eight patients (3%) submitted to an AR, the onset of DM was observed in two cases after middle pancreatectomy. No differences were found in terms of DM rate between patients who developed high-grade vs. low-grade or no postoperative complications ($p = 0.647$). Among those nine patients who underwent islet autotransplatation, the onset of DM was observed in four cases. All these four patients had a BMI greater than 25 Kg/m^2 (in three out of four cases BMI was greater than 30 Kg/m^2). None of the patients submitted to islet autotransplatation developed complications related to the procedure. At multivariate logistic regression analysis (Table 3), a BMI that was greater than 25 Kg/m^2 was the only independent predictor of postoperative DM (Odds Ratio (OR) 4.945, 95% Confidence Interval (C.I.) 1.889–12.943, $p = 0.001$). The rates of DM in normal-weight, overweight, and obese patients were 8%, 32%, and 38%, respectively. Among male patients with a BMI greater than 25 Kg/m^2, the development of postoperative DM was observed in 40% of cases. This rate increased to 50% when the study population was stratified while using 28 Kg/m^2 as BMI cut-off.

Table 2. Comparison of demographic, clinical and pathological characteristics between patients submitted to surgery for pancreatic neuroendocrine neoplasms (PanNEN) who developed postoperative diabetes mellitus (DM) ($n = 68$) and those who did not ($n = 208$).

Variable	Total Population $n = 276$	No Postoperative DM $n = 210$	Postoperative DM $n = 68$	p Value
Age, years	58 (49;67)	56 (46;67)	60 (56;67)	**0.002**
Gender				
Male	138 (50)	95 (46)	43 (63)	
Female	138 (50)	113 (54)	25 (37)	**0.017**
Preoperative BMI, Kg/m^2	25 (22;27)	24 (22;27)	27 (25;30)	**<0.0001**
PanNEN functionality				
Nonfunctioning	225 (82)	163 (78)	62 (91)	
Functioning	51 (18)	45 (22)	6 (9)	**0.019**
Inherited Syndrome				
No	261 (95)	194 (93)	67 (99)	
Yes	15 (5)	14 (7)	1 (1)	0.127
Type of Surgery				
Pancreaticoduodenectomy	76 (27)	61 (29)	15 (22)	
Distal Pancreatectomy	192 (70)	141 (68)	51 (75)	
Atypical Resection	8 (3)	6 (3)	2 (3)	0.476
T stage [28]				
T1–T2	180 (65)	136 (65)	44 (65)	
T3–T4	96 (35)	72 (35)	24 (35)	0.919
Tumor grade [3]				
G1	153 (55)	110 (53)	43 (63)	
G2	110 (40)	85 (41)	25 (37)	
G3	13 (5)	13 (6)	0 (0)	0.065
Complications [26]				
No-I-II	239 (87)	179 (85)	60 (88)	
III-IV	37 (13)	29 (15)	8 (12)	0.647

BMI: Body Mass Index; PanNEN: Pancreatic Neuroendocrine Neoplasm; Data are expressed as number (%) or interquartile range (IQR).

Table 3. Multivariate logistic regression analysis of predictors of postoperative diabetes mellitus (DM).

Variable	OR	95% C.I.	p
Gender			
Male	1	-	
Female	0.481	0.178–1.305	0.151
Age			
≤60 years	1	-	
>60 years	0.972	0.366–2.579	0.954
Preoperative BMI			
≤25 Kg/m^2	1	-	
>25 Kg/m^2	4.945	1.889–12.943	**0.001**
Type of PanNEN			
Nonfunctioning	1	-	
Functioning	0.269	0.071–1.022	0.054

BMI: Body Mass Index; PanNEN: Pancreatic Neuroendocrine Neoplasm.

3.3. Postoperative PEI

Overall, 118 patients (43%) developed a postoperative PEI. Table 4 reports a comparison of demographic, perioperative, and pathological characteristics between patients who developed PEI and those who did not. The onset of PEI was significantly more frequent after PD when compared to DP and atypical resections ($p < 0.0001$) as well as in patients that were diagnosed with T3–T4 tumors as compared to patients with T1–T2 tumors ($p = 0.001$). Among the eight patients (3%) who underwent an AR, the appearance of postoperative PEI was observed in two cases ($n = 1$ middle pancreatectomy, $n = 1$ middle-preserving pancreatectomy). Median preoperative BMI in patients with a diagnosis of postoperative PEI was 24 Kg/m^2 (IQR 22;25 Kg/m^2) as compared to 25 Kg/m^2 (IQR 23;28 Kg/m^2) ($p = 0.005$). Male patients with a BMI that was greater than 25 Kg/m^2 developed PEI in 20% of cases. Patients who developed high-grade postoperative complications (Clavien-Dindo III-IV) displayed a higher frequency of PEI ($p = 0.027$). At multivariate logistic regression analysis (Table 5) pancreaticoduodenectomy was the only independent predictor of postoperative pancreatic exocrine insufficiency onset (OR 31.680; 95% CI 10.622–94.487; $p < 0.0001$).

Table 4. Comparison of demographic, clinical and pathological characteristics between patients submitted to surgery for pancreatic neuroendocrine neoplasms (PanNEN) who developed postoperative pancreatic exocrine insufficiency (PEI) (n = 118) and those who did not (n = 158).

Variable	Total Population n = 276	No Postoperative PEI n = 158	Postoperative PEI n = 118	p Value
Age, years	58 (49;67)	58 (49;65)	60 (47;68)	0.556
Gender				
Male	138 (50)	76 (48)	62 (53)	
Female	138 (50)	82 (52)	56 (47)	0.543
BMI, Kg/m^2	24.5 (22.5;27)	25 (23;28)	24 (22;25)	**0.005**
Type of PanNEN				
Non-functioning	225 (82)	123 (78)	102 (86)	
Functioning	51 (18)	35 (22)	16 (14)	0.085
Inherited Syndrome				
No	261 (95)	150 (95)	111 (94)	
Yes	15 (5)	8 (5)	7 (6)	0.793
Type of Surgery				
Pancreaticoduodenectomy	76 (27)	8 (5)	68 (58)	
Distal Pancreatectomy	192 (70)	144 (91)	48 (41)	
Atypical Resection	8 (3)	6 (4)	2 (1)	**<0.0001**
T stage [28]				
T1–T2	180 (65)	116 (73)	64 (54)	
T3–T4	96 (35)	42 (27)	54 (46)	**0.001**
Tumor grade [3]				
G1	153 (55)	96 (61)	57 (48)	
G2	110 (40)	55 (35)	55 (47)	
G3	13 (5)	7 (4)	6 (5)	0.108
Complications [26]				
No-I-II	239 (87)	143 (91)	96 (81)	
III-IV	37 (13)	15 (9)	22 (19)	**0.027**

BMI: Body Mass Index; PanNEN: Pancreatic Neuroendocrine neoplasm; Data are expressed as number (%) or median (interquartile range (IQR)).

Table 5. Multivariate logistic regression analysis of predictors of postoperative pancreatic exocrine insufficiency.

Variable	OR	95% C.I.	p
BMI			
≤25 Kg/m^2	1	-	
>25 Kg/m^2	0.746	0.280–1.989	0.558
Type of Surgery			
Distal Pancreatectomy	1	-	
Pancreaticoduodenectomy	31.68	10.622–94.487	**<0.0001**
Atypical resection	4.8	0.626–36.818	0.131
T stage [28]			
T1–T2	1	-	
T3–T4	1.245	0.461–3.365	0.665
Complications [26]			
No-I–II	1	-	
III–IV	1.464	0.330–6.486	0.616

BMI: Body Mass Index.

3.4. Long-Term Oncological Outcomes

After a median follow-up of 72 months (IQR 38;103 months), 54 patients (20%) developed a disease recurrence, and 22 (8%) eventually died of disease. Overall, 11 patients (4%) died for other causes that were not tumor-related. The overall PFS and OS rates at five years were 80% and 91%, respectively. The effect of postoperative DM and PEI was then tested against PFS, whereas it was not tested against OS, since the number of disease-specific deaths was too low. No statistically significant differences were found in terms of PFS between patients with and without postoperative DM (five-year PFS rate 80% vs. 80%, $p = 0.827$). Patients without PEI had better PFS when compared to patients who developed a postoperative PEI (five-year PFS rate 86% vs. 71%, $p = 0.002$). At multivariate analysis, adjusted for age, gender, T stage, N stage, M stage, grading, microvascular invasion, perineural invasion, and necrosis, postoperative exocrine pancreatic insufficiency was no longer a predictor of disease recurrence/progression (Hazard Ratio (HR) 1.497; 95% CI 0.840–2.669; $p = 0.171$).

4. Discussion

PanNEN have a more indolent biological behaviour and they are usually associated to a longer survival when compared to their exocrine counterpart. Therefore, it is of paramount importance to evaluate the long-term functional sequelae following pancreatic resection for PanNEN and to find a balance between the oncological risk and the impact of endocrine and exocrine impairment on general health status. Various studies have explored the functional outcomes after pancreatic resection in large populations, including patients affected by different pancreatic diseases, ranging from benign conditions to cancer [19,20,29–31]. In contrast, data on the long-term endocrine and exocrine pancreatic insufficiency after pancreatic surgery specifically performed for PanNEN are currently limited [32]. The risk of developing a postoperative DM and/or PEI can be influenced by specific characteristics that are related to the underlying primary pancreatic disease.

The incidence of post-pancreatectomy DM ranges from 5% to 78% [20,30,31,33,34], probably due to the heterogeneity of the selecting criteria of study populations and to the different duration of follow-up. In the present series, the onset of postoperative DM was observed in nearly one-third of patients after six years from surgery. A similar incidence of DM (23%) was reported in a series including 229 patients submitted to surgery for benign tumors [20]. In contrast, the incidence reported by Falconi et al. [19] in a previous study including only benign diseases was lower, with postoperative DM being reported only in the 14% of cases after DP and in the 18% of cases after PD, respectively [19]. Similarly, another series, including only benign or low-grade malignant neoplasms, reported a low incidence of postoperative DM (<10%) after a median follow-up of less than two years [35]. The higher incidence of DM found in the present series is probably related to the longer duration of follow-up, which also represents one of the main strengths of the present study. Various factors have been described as being able to influence the risk of developing endocrine insufficiency: these include the extent of resection, the nature of disease, some patient's characteristics, and the functionality of the remaining parenchyma [19].

In the present series, BMI was found to be the only independent predictor of postoperative DM: specifically, a BMI greater than 25 Kg/m^2 increased the risk of developing postoperative DM up to five times. Of note, four out of nine patients submitted to islet autotransplantation developed postoperative DM: all of them had a BMI greater than 25 Kg/m^2. This result corroborates previous findings reporting that increasing BMI is associated to a higher risk of postoperative endocrine insufficiency [20,29,36]. This result confirms the importance of a personalised prehabilitation before surgery in those patients who are overweight or obese. At this regard, the relatively indolent nature of PanNEN allows for safely postponing the day of operation from initial diagnosis. The result here presented is consistent with data from the National Health and Nutrition Examination Surgery (NAHNES) reporting that the prevalence of DM in general population increases with the increasing of BMI class [37]. According to this survey, the prevalence of DM among normal-weight patients is around 8%, whereas it is reported to almost double (15%) in the overweight patients. The prevalence of DM increases even more in obese patients, attesting itself around 28% [37]. In the present series, overweight patients developed postoperative DM in 32% of cases (vs. 15% in general population), whereas the rate of DM among obese patients was 38% (vs. 28% in general population). In contrast, normal-weight patients developed postoperative DM in 8% of cases, consistently with data that were reported in general population. Moreover, patients who developed a postoperative DM were more frequently males and had an older age compared to those who did not. Although these findings were not confirmed at multivariate analysis, they represent well-known risk factors for DM and they were also reported by other series as factors that are associated to the development of postoperative DM [19,29]. In particular, according to data from the Study to Help Improve Early evaluation and management of risk factors Leading to Diabetes (SHIELD), male patients with a high BMI ($\geq$ 28 Kg/m^2) display a DM prevalence of around 40%, whereas in the present series half of patients with the same characteristics developed DM, which suggested that the pancreatic resection has a role in determining the onset of the disease. Interestingly, no statistically significant differences were found in terms of risk of developing DM between patients submitted to different surgical procedures, even if a trend towards a higher incidence of DM after DP (26%) than after PD (20%) was observed, as previously reported by other series [20,29]. Probably, in the present series, the difference between DP and PD failed to reach a statistically significant difference because patients that were submitted to DP had smaller tumors when compared to patients who underwent PD. Consequently, the extent of DP was often limited for sparing parenchyma and preserving its functionality. Various studies have previously reported a lower incidence of postoperative pancreatic impairment after parenchyma-sparing surgery [15,17–19]. In the present series, patients that were submitted to enucleation were excluded in order to focus on partial pancreatic resections; therefore, as only eight patients submitted to atypical resections (middle pancreatectomy or middle-preserving pancreatectomy) were considered, a statistically significant difference in terms of DM development between these subjects and those that were submitted to a formal resection could not be demonstrated. However, when patients also submitted to enucleation were considered for this specific analysis, the rate of postoperative DM was significantly lower ($p = 0.001$) in those that were submitted to a parenchyma-sparing surgery (10%) when compared to those who underwent a formal resection (25%).

The occurrence of PEI is another important outcome following pancreatic resection [7]. PEI is frequently misdiagnosed, as it usually presents with mild or moderate symptoms that may be underestimated, leading to a poor quality of life [8], micronutrients deficiencies [38] and decreased survival [10]. In the present study, the overall incidence of PEI was 43% that is consistent with the rate reported by Lim et al. [39]. The rate of PEI development that was reported in literature varies between 56% and 98% after PD [7,8,40] and between 19% and 80% after DP [7]. This wide range is probably due to the different methods that were used to assess pancreatic exocrine function and to the low accuracy of available tests in determining PEI [41]. Of note, in the present series, exocrine impairment was observed in nearly nine out of 10 patients after PD and this operation was found to be independently associated with an increased risk of PEI. PD has been widely demonstrated to be strongly correlated to PEI [29,39,42]. The higher frequency of PEI after PD is essentially explained by the surgical reconstruction, as it can predispose to a progressive damage of the remaining pancreatic stump [43], to bile salt malabsorption [44] and to bacterial overgrowth [7]. In the present series, a lower rate of PEI among patients submitted to atypical resection could not be demonstrated, as only eight patients undergoing this kind of surgery were included. However, when also patients submitted to enucleation were considered for this specific analysis, the rate of PEI after parenchyma-sparing surgery was significantly lower (2%) than after formal resection (43%). Moreover, a lower preoperative BMI was found to be associated with a higher rate of PEI, as previously reported by Kusakabe et al. [29]. At this regard, it is possible that patients with a lower preoperative BMI have an undiagnosed preoperative PEI and, consequently, they are more likely to develop an evident PEI after pancreatic resection. Finally, patients who developed high-grade postoperative complications displayed a significantly higher rate of PEI when compared to other patients. However, this association was not confirmed at multivariate analysis, probably because patients with high-grade postoperative complications were the same who underwent PD, which is an independent predictor of PEI development.

Our findings are in partial agreement with the few previous reports that were obtained in smaller series. Neophytou et al. [32] investigated the postoperative rate of DM and PEI in 92 patients operated for benign tumours, including PanNEN. Factors that were associated with the occurrence of DM were male sex, a BMI > 28 Kg/m^2 and metabolic syndrome, whereas factors that were associated with the risk of PEI were preoperative chronic pancreatitis, a BMI < 18.5 Kg/m^2 and tumors located in the pancreatic head. Of note, although the role of chronic pancreatitis in the remnant pancreas was not investigated, this is unlikely to be relevant in PanNEN, as patients who undergo pancreatic resection for these neoplasms usually have a normal, non-fibrotic, pancreatic remnant that was not affected by the presence of the tumor. Indeed, PanNEN typically exhibit an expansive evolution rather than an infiltrative growth.

In the present series, DM occurred as a gradual phenomenon, as the majority of patients did not develop it immediately after surgery, but during follow up, over the course of several months or even years, consistently with data that were previously reported by Falconi et al. [19]. This finding corroborates the fact that the development of DM is not only dependent from the surgical procedure, but even after a pancreatic resection, other factors, such as a BMI > 25 Kg/m^2, strongly contribute to its appearance. In contrast, most of patients developed PEI in the early postoperative period, probably because its occurrence is strictly related to the surgical procedure. As previously pointed out, PD is more frequently associated with PEI and its early occurrence might be related not only to the reduced pancreatic volume, but also to a sudden impairment of pancreatic stimulation, which is physiologically induced by endocrine cells of the resected duodenum [43]. However, one could speculate that patients that were submitted to PD could experience a worsening of PEI during follow up as the surgical reconstruction associated to PD can predispose to progressive damage and atrophy of the pancreatic stump.

The secondary outcome of the present study was to investigate whether endocrine or exocrine pancreatic insufficiency were associated with disease outcome. We focused on the association with PFS, as the rate of disease-related deaths was low, as expected for surgically treated PanNEN. While DM was not associated with PFS, there was a lower five-year PFS rate in patients who developed PEI. However, when corrected for other prognostic factors at multivariate regression, PEI was not a significant factor.

The overall rate of postoperative DM and PEI observed in the present series is relatively high (24% and 43% for DM and PEI, respectively), and it has been reported that pancreatic impairment might be associated with a significant impact on general health status and on quality of life [7,8]. This is one of the reasons in support of an active surveillance management instead of a pancreatic resection for patients that were affected by non-functioning PanNEN ≤ 2 cm without features of aggressiveness [6,45,46].

The present study has several limitations. The major limit is represented by the retrospective design. Secondly, the diagnosis of PEI was not based on specific tests objectively evaluating the pancreatic function, but on the presence of related signs and symptoms that were cured with pancreatic enzymes replacement treatment. However, the accuracy and feasibility of the available tests are currently debated [41]. Indirect tests, such as fecal elastase-1, fecal chymotrypsin, and 13C breath test, evaluate the quantitative changes of pancreatic secretion and are less expensive, easier to be performed, but less accurate, compared to direct ones. Direct tests, on the contrary, evaluate directly the secretive production, but, despite their good sensitivity, are invasive, time-consuming, and expensive [41]. However, the use of both these test after pancreatic surgery is unreliable. Indeed, it has been reported that fecal elastase 1 is not accurate in diagnosing PEI after pancreatic surgery [47]. 13C breath test has been previously performed to evaluate pancreatic exocrine function in patients that were submitted to pancreatic resection [48,49] and it seems to be more accurate than fecal elastase-1 [48]. However, the validity of 13C breath test is still questionable as a comparison between this test and a gold standard (72 h fecal fats or bicarbonate dosage in pancreatic juice) in patients that were submitted to pancreatic surgery has not been made. Of note, when PD is performed, besides the reduced enzyme output following the removal of pancreatic parenchyma, other factors, such as small bowel bacterial overgrowth, deranged antral grinding, abnormal mixing of food with digestive secretions, abnormal hormonal stimulation, and acidic intraluminal pH, can affect the results [47]. Moreover, various steps, including gastric emptying time of the tracer, absorption, hepatic circulation, and metabolism, are involved in breath test and some of them might be altered after pancreatic resection [48]. Regarding direct tests, such as endoscopic aspiration of pancreatic juice, it has to be said that they are invasive and cannot be performed when anatomy is modified by surgical procedures [40]. Another possible limitation of the present study is represented by the lack of data on the possible role of medical treatments initiated during follow-up for a recurrence of the PanNET, which might have contributed to occurrence of PEI [50]. However, the rate of PEI occurring after tumor recurrence was 54% in patients that were treated with somatostatin analogues and 69% in patients who did not us them, which suggests that this is not a relevant issue. Finally, a more complete analysis of pancreatic endocrine function with the execution of oral glucose tolerance test (OGTT), dosage of insulin and C-peptide, and calculation of Homeostatic Model Assessment for Insulin Resistance (HOMA-IR) could have been performed, thus adding interesting information regarding glucose metabolism in patients that were submitted to pancreatic resection. However, according to the current American Diabetes Association (ADA) guidelines, either fasting plasma glucose (FPG), 2-h plasma glucose during 75 g OGTT and HbA1c are equally appropriate for diagnosing DM [23]. In particular, HbA1c seems to have some advantages when compared to both FPG and OGTT, as it is reported to have a greater convenience (as fasting is not required), a greater pre-analytical stability, and fewer perturbations during stress and illness [23]. This is an important point given the fact that patients who undergo a pancreatic resection are subjected to a severe physical stress, which could easily alter plasma glucose levels.

In conclusion, the present study demonstrated that the risk of postoperative pancreatic endocrine and exocrine insufficiency after surgery for PanNEN is significantly high and patients should be aware of these complications. A personalized prehabilitation should be recommended in those patients with a BMI > 25 kg/m^2 for reducing the risk of DM development in the postoperative period. Endocrine and exocrine insufficiency do not seem to influence PFS. Further studies are needed to better elucidate the time of onset and the severity of DM and/or PEI and to assess their impact on quality of life of patients that were surgically treated for PanNEN.

Author Contributions: Conceptualization, V.A., S.P. and M.F.; Formal analysis, V.A. and S.P.; Investigation, V.A. and F.M.; Project administration, M.F.; Supervision, S.P. and Gabriele Capurso; Writing—original draft, V.A., S.P. and G.C.; Writing—review & editing, G.B., S.C. and M.F. All the authors have approved the submitted version and agree to be personally accountable for the author's own contributions and for ensuring that questions related to the accuracy or integrity of any part of the work are appropriately investigated, resolved, and documented in the literature.

Acknowledgments: Valentina Andreasi studentship and Francesca Muffatti research fellowship were supported by Gioja Bianca Costanza legacy donation.

Conflicts of Interest: The authors declare no conflict of interest.

References

1. Dasari, A.; Shen, C.; Halperin, D.; Zhao, B.; Zhou, S.; Xu, Y.; Shih, T.; Yao, J.C. Trends in the Incidence, Prevalence, and Survival Outcomes in Patients With Neuroendocrine Tumors in the United States. *JAMA Oncol.* **2017**, *3*, 1335–1342. [CrossRef] [PubMed]
2. Kuo, E.J.; Salem, R.R. Population-level analysis of pancreatic neuroendocrine tumors 2 cm or less in size. *Ann. Surg. Oncol.* **2013**, *20*, 2815–2821. [CrossRef] [PubMed]
3. Lloyd, R.V.; Osamura, R.Y.; Kloppel, G.; Rosai, J. *WHO Classification of Tumours of Endocrine Organs*, 4th ed.; Lloyd, R.V., Osamura, R.Y., Kloppel, G., Rosai, J., Eds.; IARC Press: Lyon, France, 2017.
4. Partelli, S.; Javed, A.A.; Andreasi, V.; He, J.; Muffatti, F.; Weiss, M.J.; Sessa, F.; La Rosa, S.; Doglioni, C.; Zamboni, G.; et al. The number of positive nodes accurately predicts recurrence after pancreaticoduodenectomy for nonfunctioning neuroendocrine neoplasms. *Eur. J. Surg. Oncol.* **2018**, *44*, 778–783. [CrossRef] [PubMed]
5. Genc, C.G.; Jilesen, A.P.; Partelli, S.; Falconi, M.; Muffatti, F.; van Kemenade, F.J.; van Eeden, S.; Verheij, J.; van Dieren, S.; van Eijck, C.H.J.; et al. A New Scoring System to Predict Recurrent Disease in Grade 1 and 2 Nonfunctional Pancreatic Neuroendocrine Tumors. *Ann. Surg.* **2018**, *267*, 1148–1154. [CrossRef]
6. Falconi, M.; Eriksson, B.; Kaltsas, G.; Bartsch, D.K.; Capdevila, J.; Caplin, M.; Kos-Kudla, B.; Kwekkeboom, D.; Rindi, G.; Kloppel, G.; et al. ENETS Consensus Guidelines Update for the Management of Patients with Functional Pancreatic Neuroendocrine Tumors and Non-Functional Pancreatic Neuroendocrine Tumors. *Neuroendocrinology* **2016**, *103*, 153–171. [CrossRef]
7. Phillips, M.E. Pancreatic exocrine insufficiency following pancreatic resection. *Pancreatology* **2015**, *15*, 449–455. [CrossRef]
8. Halloran, C.M.; Cox, T.F.; Chauhan, S.; Raraty, M.G.T.; Sutton, R.; Neoptolemos, J.P.; Ghaneh, P. Partial pancreatic resection for pancreatic malignancy is associated with sustained pancreatic exocrine failure and reduced quality of life: A prospective study. *Pancreatology* **2011**, *11*, 535–545. [CrossRef]
9. Armstrong, T.; Strommer, L.; Ruiz-Jasbon, F.; Shek, F.W.; Harris, S.F.; Permert, J.; Johnson, C.D. Pancreaticoduodenectomy for peri-ampullary neoplasia leads to specific micronutrient deficiencies. *Pancreatology* **2007**, *7*, 37–44. [CrossRef]
10. Winny, M.; Paroglou, V.; Bektas, H.; Kaltenborn, A.; Reichert, B.; Zachau, L.; Kleine, M.; Klempnauer, J.; Schrem, H. Insulin dependence and pancreatic enzyme replacement therapy are independent prognostic factors for long-term survival after operation for chronic pancreatitis. *Surg. (U. S.)* **2014**, *155*, 271–279. [CrossRef]
11. Iacono, C.; Verlato, G.; Ruzzenente, A.; Campagnaro, T.; Bacchelli, C.; Valdegamberi, A.; Bortolasi, L.; Guglielmi, A. Systematic review of central pancreatectomy and meta-analysis of central versus distal pancreatectomy. *Br. J. Surg.* **2013**, *100*, 873–885. [CrossRef]
12. Santangelo, M.; Esposito, A.; Tammaro, V.; Calogero, A.; Criscitiello, C.; Roberti, G.; Candida, M.; Rupealta, N.; Pisani, A.; Carlomagno, N. What indication, morbidity and mortality for central pancreatectomy in oncological surgery? A systematic review. *Int. J. Surg.* **2016**, *28*, 172–176. [CrossRef] [PubMed]
13. Beger, H.G.; Siech, M.; Poch, B.; Mayer, B.; Schoenberg, M.H. Limited surgery for benign tumours of the pancreas: A systematic review. *World J. Surg.* **2015**, *39*, 1557–1566. [CrossRef] [PubMed]
14. Gharios, J.; Hain, E.; Dohan, A.; Prat, F.; Terris, B.; Bertherat, J.; Coriat, R.; Dousset, B.; Gaujoux, S. Pre- and intraoperative diagnostic requirements, benefits and risks of minimally invasive and robotic surgery for neuroendocrine tumors of the pancreas. *Best Pract. Res. Clin. Endocrinol. Metab.* **2019**. [CrossRef] [PubMed]

15. Crippa, S.; Bassi, C.; Salvia, R.; Falconi, M.; Butturini, G.; Pederzoli, P. Enucleation of pancreatic neoplasms. *Br. J. Surg.* **2007**, *94*, 1254–1259. [CrossRef] [PubMed]
16. Cauley, C.E.; Pitt, H.A.; Ziegler, K.M.; Nakeeb, A.; Schmidt, C.M.; Zyromski, N.J.; House, M.G.; Lillemoe, K.D. Pancreatic Enucleation: Improved Outcomes Compared to Resection. *J. Gastrointest. Surg.* **2012**, *16*, 1347–1353. [CrossRef]
17. Paiella, S.; De Pastena, M.; Faustini, F.; Landoni, L.; Pollini, T.; Bonamini, D.; Giuliani, T.; Bassi, C.; Esposito, A.; Tuveri, M.; et al. Central pancreatectomy for benign or low-grade malignant pancreatic lesions—A single-center retrospective analysis of 116 cases. *Eur. J. Surg. Oncol.* **2019**, *45*, 788–792. [CrossRef]
18. Falconi, M.; Zerbi, A.; Crippa, S.; Balzano, G.; Boninsegna, L.; Capitanio, V.; Bassi, C.; Di Carlo, V.; Pederzoli, P. Parenchyma-Preserving resections for small nonfunctioning pancreatic endocrine tumors. *Ann. Surg. Oncol.* **2010**, *17*, 1621–1627. [CrossRef]
19. Falconi, M.; Mantovani, W.; Crippa, S.; Mascetta, G.; Salvia, R.; Pederzoli, P. Pancreatic insufficiency after different resections for benign tumours. *Br. J. Surg.* **2008**, *95*, 85–91. [CrossRef]
20. Kwon, J.H.; Kim, S.C.; Shim, I.K.; Song, K.B.; Lee, J.H.; Hwang, D.W.; Park, K.M.; Lee, Y.J. Factors affecting the development of diabetes mellitus after pancreatic resection. *Pancreas* **2015**, *44*, 1296–1303. [CrossRef]
21. Malka, D.; Hammel, P.; Sauvanet, A.; Rufat, P. Risk factors for diabetes mellitus in chronic pancreatitis. *Gastroenterology* **2000**, *119*, 1324–1332. [CrossRef]
22. Von Elm, E.; Altman, D.G.; Egger, M.; Pocock, S.J.; Gotzsche, P.C.; Vandenbroucke, J.P. The Strengthening the Reporting of Observational Studies in Epidemiology (STROBE) Statement: Guidelines for reporting observational studies. *Int. J. Surg.* **2014**, *12*, 1495–1499. [CrossRef] [PubMed]
23. American Diabetes Association. 2. Classification and Diagnosis of Diabetes: Standards of Medical Care in Diabetes-2019. *Diabetes Care* **2019**, *42*, 13–28. [CrossRef] [PubMed]
24. Partelli, S.; Boninsegna, L.; Salvia, R.; Bassi, C.; Pederzoli, P.; Falconi, M. Middle-preserving pancreatectomy for multicentric body-sparing lesions of the pancreas. *Am. J. Surg.* **2009**, *198*, 49–53. [CrossRef]
25. Balzano, G.; Maffi, P.; Nano, R.; Mercalli, A.; Melzi, R.; Aleotti, F.; Zerbi, A.; De Cobelli, F.; Gavazzi, F.; Magistretti, P.; et al. Autologous Islet Transplantation in Patients Requiring Pancreatectomy: A Broader Spectrum of Indications Beyond Chronic Pancreatitis. *Am. J. Transplant.* **2016**, *16*, 1812–1826. [CrossRef] [PubMed]
26. Dindo, D.; Demartines, N.; Clavien, P.-A. Classification of surgical complications: A new proposal with evaluation in a cohort of 6336 patients and results of a survey. *Ann. Surg.* **2004**, *240*, 205–213. [CrossRef] [PubMed]
27. Bassi, C.; Marchegiani, G.; Dervenis, C.; Sarr, M.; Abu Hilal, M.; Adham, M.; Allen, P.; Andersson, R.; Asbun, H.J.; Besselink, M.G.; et al. The 2016 update of the International Study Group (ISGPS) definition and grading of postoperative pancreatic fistula: 11 Years After. *Surgery* **2017**, *161*, 584–591. [CrossRef] [PubMed]
28. Rindi, G.; Kloppel, G.; Couvelard, A.; Komminoth, P.; Korner, M.; Lopes, J.M.; McNicol, A.-M.; Nilsson, O.; Perren, A.; Scarpa, A.; et al. TNM staging of midgut and hindgut (neuro) endocrine tumors: A consensus proposal including a grading system. *Virchows Arch.* **2007**, *451*, 757–762. [CrossRef]
29. Kusakabe, J.; Anderson, B.; Liu, J.; Williams, G.A.; Chapman, W.C.; Doyle, M.M.B.; Khan, A.S.; Sanford, D.E.; Hammill, C.W.; Strasberg, S.M.; et al. Long-Term Endocrine and Exocrine Insufficiency After Pancreatectomy. *J. Gastrointest. Surg.* **2019**, *23*, 1604–1613. [CrossRef]
30. Shirakawa, S.; Matsumoto, I.; Toyama, H.; Shinzeki, M.; Ajiki, T.; Fukumoto, T.; Ku, Y. Pancreatic Volumetric Assessment as a Predictor of New-Onset Diabetes Following Distal Pancreatectomy. *J. Gastrointest. Surg.* **2012**, *16*, 2212–2219. [CrossRef]
31. You, D.D.; Choi, S.H.; Choi, D.W.; Heo, J.S.; Ho, C.Y.; Kim, W.S. Long-term effects of pancreaticoduodenectomy on glucose metabolism. *ANZ J. Surg.* **2012**, *82*, 447–451. [CrossRef]
32. Neophytou, H.; Wangermez, M.; Gand, E.; Carretier, M.; Danion, J.; Richer, J.-P. Predictive factors of endocrine and exocrine insufficiency after resection of a benign tumour of the pancreas. *Ann. Endocrinol. (Paris)* **2018**, *79*, 53–61. [CrossRef] [PubMed]
33. King, J.; Kazanjian, K.; Matsumoto, J.; Reber, H.A.; Yeh, M.W.; Hines, O.J.; Eibl, G. Distal pancreatectomy: Incidence of postoperative diabetes. *J. Gastrointest. Surg.* **2008**, *12*, 1548–1553. [CrossRef] [PubMed]
34. Lee, S.E.; Jang, J.Y.; Hwang, D.W.; Lee, K.U.; Kim, S.W. Clinical efficacy of organ-preserving pancreatectomy for benign or low-grade malignant potential lesion. *J. Korean Med. Sci.* **2010**, *25*, 97–103. [CrossRef] [PubMed]

35. Shoup, M.; Brennan, M.F.; McWhite, K.; Leung, D.H.Y.; Klimstra, D.; Conlon, K.C. The value of splenic preservation with distal pancreatectomy. *Arch. Surg.* **2002**, *137*, 164–168. [CrossRef]
36. Hirata, K.; Nakata, B.; Amano, R.; Yamazoe, S.; Kimura, K.; Hirakawa, K. Predictive Factors for Change of Diabetes Mellitus Status After Pancreatectomy in Preoperative Diabetic and Nondiabetic Patients. *J. Gastrointest. Surg.* **2014**, *18*, 1597–1603. [CrossRef]
37. Nguyen, N.T.; Nguyen, X.M.T.; Lane, J.; Wang, P. Relationship between obesity and diabetes in a US adult population: Findings from the national health and nutrition examination survey, 1999–2006. *Obes. Surg.* **2011**, *21*, 351–355. [CrossRef]
38. Mann, S.T.W.; Stracke, H.; Lange, U.; Klör, H.U.; Teichmann, J. Vitamin D3 in patients with various grades of chronic pancreatitis, according to morphological and functional criteria of the pancreas. *Dig. Dis. Sci.* **2003**, *48*, 533–538. [CrossRef]
39. Lim, P.W.; Dinh, K.H.; Sullivan, M.; Wassef, W.Y.; Zivny, J.; Whalen, G.F.; LaFemina, J. Thirty-day outcomes underestimate endocrine and exocrine insufficiency after pancreatic resection. *HPB* **2016**, *18*, 360–366. [CrossRef]
40. Matsumoto, J.; Traverso, L.W. Exocrine Function Following the Whipple Operation as Assessed by Stool Elastase. *J. Gastrointest. Surg.* **2006**, *10*, 1225–1229. [CrossRef]
41. Capurso, G.; Traini, M.; Piciucchi, M.; Signoretti, M.; Arcidiacono, P.G. Exocrine pancreatic insufficiency: Prevalence, diagnosis, and management. *Clin. Exp. Gastroenterol.* **2019**, *12*, 129–139. [CrossRef]
42. Kachare, S.D.; Fitzgerald, T.L.; Schuth, O.; Vohra, N.A.; Zervos, E.E. The impact of pancreatic resection on exocrine homeostasis. *Am. Surg.* **2014**, *80*, 704–709. [PubMed]
43. Benini, L.; Gabbrielli, A.; Cristofori, C.; Amodio, A.; Butturini, G.; Cardobi, N.; Sozzi, C.; Frulloni, L.; Mucelli, R.P.; Crinò, S.; et al. Residual pancreatic function after pancreaticoduodenectomy is better preserved with pancreaticojejunostomy than pancreaticogastrostomy: A long-term analysis. *Pancreatology* **2019**, *9*, 595–601. [CrossRef] [PubMed]
44. Tran, T.C.K.; Van Lanschot, J.J.B.; Bruno, M.J.; Van Eijck, C.H.J. Functional changes after pancreatoduodenectomy: Diagnosis and treatment. *Pancreatology* **2009**, *9*, 729–737. [CrossRef] [PubMed]
45. Bettini, R.; Partelli, S.; Boninsegna, L.; Capelli, P.; Crippa, S.; Pederzoli, P.; Scarpa, A.; Falconi, M. Tumor size correlates with malignancy in nonfunctioning pancreatic endocrine tumor. *Surgery* **2011**, *150*, 75–82. [CrossRef] [PubMed]
46. Gaujoux, S.; Partelli, S.; Maire, F.; D'Onofrio, M.; Larroque, B.; Tamburrino, D.; Sauvanet, A.; Falconi, M.; Ruszniewski, P. Observational study of natural history of small sporadic nonfunctioning pancreatic neuroendocrine tumors. *J. Clin. Endocrinol. Metab.* **2013**, *98*, 4784–4789. [CrossRef] [PubMed]
47. Benini, L.; Amodio, A.; Campagnola, P.; Agugiaro, F.; Cristofori, C.; Micciolo, R.; Magro, A.; Gabbrielli, A.; Cabrini, G.; Moser, L.; et al. Fecal elastase-1 is useful in the detection of steatorrhea in patients with pancreatic diseases but not after pancreatic resection. *Pancreatology* **2013**, *13*, 38–42. [CrossRef] [PubMed]
48. Nakamura, H.; Morifuji, M.; Murakami, Y.; Uemura, K.; Ohge, H.; Hayashidani, Y.; Sudo, T.; Sueda, T. Usefulness of a 13C-labeled mixed triglyceride breath test for assessing pancreatic exocrine function after pancreatic surgery. *Surgery* **2009**, *145*, 168–175. [CrossRef] [PubMed]
49. Alfieri, S.; Agnes, A.; Rosa, F.; Di Miceli, D.; Grieco, D.L.; Scaldaferri, F.; Gasbarrini, A.; Doglietto, G.B.; Quero, G. Long-term pancreatic exocrine and endometabolic functionality after pancreaticoduodenectomy. Comparison between pancreaticojejunostomy and pancreatic duct occlusion with fibrin glue. *Eur. Rev. Med. Pharmacol. Sci.* **2018**, *22*, 4310–4318.
50. Lamarca, A.; McCallum, L.; Nuttall, C.; Barriuso, J.; Backen, A.; Frizziero, M.; Leon, R.; Mansoor, W.; McNamara, M.G.; Hubner, R.A.; et al. Somatostatin analogue-induced pancreatic exocrine insufficiency in patients with neuroendocrine tumors: Results of a prospective observational study. *Expert Rev. Gastroenterol. Hepatol.* **2018**, *12*, 723–731. [CrossRef]

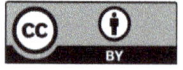

© 2019 by the authors. Licensee MDPI, Basel, Switzerland. This article is an open access article distributed under the terms and conditions of the Creative Commons Attribution (CC BY) license (http://creativecommons.org/licenses/by/4.0/).

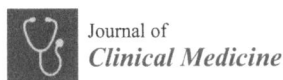

Article

Consensus-Derived Quality Performance Indicators for Neuroendocrine Tumour Care

Braden Woodhouse [1], Sharon Pattison [2], Eva Segelov [3], Simron Singh [4], Kate Parker [1], Grace Kong [5], William Macdonald [6], David Wyld [7,8], Goswin Meyer-Rochow [9], Nick Pavlakis [10], Siobhan Conroy [11], Vallerie Gordon [12], Jonathan Koea [13], Nicole Kramer [14], Michael Michael [15], Kate Wakelin [16], Tehmina Asif [17], Dorothy Lo [18], Timothy Price [19], Ben Lawrence [1,20,*] and on behalf of the Commonwealth Neuroendocrine Tumour Collaboration (CommNETs)

1. Discipline of Oncology, Faculty of Medicine and Health Sciences, The University of Auckland, Auckland 1023, New Zealand; b.woodhouse@auckland.ac.nz (B.W.); kate.parker@auckland.ac.nz (K.P.)
2. Department of Medicine, University of Otago, Dunedin 9016, New Zealand; sharon.pattison@otago.ac.nz
3. Department of Medical Oncology, Monash University and Monash Health, Melbourne 3800, Australia; eva.segelov@monash.edu
4. Department of Medical Oncology, Sunnybrook Odette Cancer Center, University of Toronto, Toronto, ON M4N 3M5, Canada; simron.singh@sunnybrook.ca
5. Department of Nuclear Medicine, Peter MacCallum Cancer Centre, Melbourne 3000, Australia; grace.kong@petermac.org
6. Department of Nuclear Medicine, Fiona Stanley Hospital, Perth 6150, Australia; william.macdonald@health.wa.gov.au
7. Department of Medical Oncology, Royal Brisbane and Women's Hospital, Brisbane 4029, Australia; david.wyld@health.qld.gov.au
8. School of Medicine, University of Queensland, Brisbane 4072, Australia
9. Department of General Surgery, Waikato Hospital, Hamilton 3204, New Zealand; win.meyer-rochow@waikatodhb.health.nz
10. Department of Medical Oncology, Royal North Shore Hospital, Sydney 2065, Australia; nick.pavlakis@sydney.edu.au
11. Unicorn Foundation New Zealand, Auckland, New Zealand; siobhan@unicornfoundation.org.nz
12. Department of Medical Oncology, Cancer Care Manitoba, Winnipeg, MB R3E 0V9, Canada; vgordon1@cancercare.mb.ca
13. Department of General Surgery, North Shore Hospital, Auckland 0620, New Zealand; jonathan.koea@waitematadhb.govt.nz
14. Department of Pathology, North Shore Hospital, Auckland 0620, New Zealand; nicole.kramer@waitematadhb.govt.nz
15. Department of Medical Oncology, Peter MacCallum Cancer Centre, Melbourne 3000, Australia; michael.michael@petermac.org
16. Unicorn Foundation, Melbourne, Australia; kate.wakelin@unicornfoundation.org.au
17. Department of Medical Oncology, Saskatchewan Cancer Agency, Saskatoon, SK S4W 0G3, Canada; tehmina.asif@saskcancer.ca
18. Department of Medical Oncology, St Joseph's Health Care, Toronto, ON M6R 1B5, Canada; dlo@stjoestoronto.ca
19. Department of Medical Oncology, The Queen Elizabeth Hospital, Adelaide 5011, Australia; timothy.price@health.sa.gov.au
20. Department of Medical Oncology, Auckland City Hospital, Auckland 1023, New Zealand
* Correspondence: b.lawrence@auckland.ac.nz

Received: 31 July 2019; Accepted: 7 September 2019; Published: 12 September 2019

Abstract: Quality performance indicators (QPIs) are used to monitor the delivery of cancer care. Neuroendocrine tumours (NETs) are a family of individually uncommon cancers that derive from neuroendocrine cells or their precursors, and can occur in most organs. There are currently no QPIs available for NETs and their heterogeneity makes QPI development difficult. CommNETs is a collaboration between NET clinicians, researchers and advocates in Canada, Australia and New

Zealand. We created QPIs for NETs using a three-step consensus process. First, a multidisciplinary team used the nominal group technique to create candidates (*n* = 133) which were then curated into appropriateness statements (62 statements, 44 sub-statements). A two-stage modified RAND/UCLA Delphi consensus process was conducted: an online survey rated the statement appropriateness then the top-ranked statements (*n* = 20) were assessed in a face-to-face meeting. Finally, 10 QPIs met consensus criteria; documentation of primary site, proliferative index, differentiation, tumour board review, use of a structured pathology report, presence of distant metastasis, 5- and 10-year disease-free and overall survival. These NET QPIs will be trialed as a method to monitor and improve care for people with NETs and to facilitate international comparison.

Keywords: quality performance indicators; QPIs; cancer care; neuroendocrine tumour; NETs; modified Delphi; CommNETs

1. Introduction

Evidence-based quality performance indicators (QPIs) are used to improve quality of cancer care by recording and publishing key aspects of each individual patient's cancer journey that contribute to outcome. For example, colorectal cancer QPIs include stoma-free survival, tumour board review, and the use of adjuvant chemotherapy [1]. QPI measurement can identify under-performing centres, and also indirectly provide standards that a service can aspire to [2–8]. QPIs have been developed in multiple countries for common malignancies such as breast or bowel cancer [1,9–12], and are usually selected from an evidence base of factors associated with outcome. This type of data are more often available in cancers that are common, have a single organ of origin (e.g., breast), and a predominant histology (e.g., adenocarcinoma). For example, separate sets of QPIs have been developed and implemented in Canada, Australia and New Zealand for colorectal cancer [1,13–17].

Neuroendocrine tumours (NETs) are a family of malignancies that derive from neuroendocrine cells or their precursors. NETs most commonly arise in the gastrointestinal tract [18], the lung and also occur in endocrine organs, thymus, skin, and all organs of the genito-urinary and gynaecological systems. Some NETs release hormones which in excess lead to specific symptoms, such as flushing and diarrhoea caused by excess serotonin secretion, or hypoglycemia caused by excess insulin, for example. Although NETs are uncommon (incidence 6.98 per 100,000), their incidence is rising [19–22], and because some NETs are very slow growing the prevalence is higher than other cancers of the same location; for example gastrointestinal NETs have a higher prevalence than pancreatic and gastric carcinomas [23].

NET outcome is highly variable by grade, usually described by proliferative index (Ki-67 and/or mitotic count), and the pace of progression varies from extremely rapid to very slow, with survival in the metastatic setting ranging from weeks to decades. Presentation will also vary due to functional status of the tumour and secreted hormone(s). This variability matters in the clinic; for example, the 5-year overall survival of rectal NETs is over 85%, whereas pancreatic NETs is less than 40% [21], and the treatments required for NETs from each site is mostly distinct. The biological heterogeneity, socioeconomic factors and regional variations of clinical care also present challenges to the treating clinical team, and present difficulties for appraising the quality of care of people with NETs within, and across health care systems [24]. QPIs that measure fundamental aspects of NET diagnosis and treatment outcome could be used to monitor the quality of NET care.

NETs present a challenge for QPI development. A QPI strategy for NETs must balance a tension between measuring fundamentals that underlie the care of all types of NETs, yet still enable detection of the variability inherent in different NET subtypes. Some pathologies that must be detected in people with NETs are very rare, thus questioning their value as a general indicator of quality care. An example is detection of carcinoid heart disease, where only a small fraction of people with NETs are affected. Types of indicators are also influenced by different healthcare systems, because data collection, regulatory processes and treatment options vary between jurisdictions. Countries like New Zealand (NZ), Canada and Australia have predominantly publically funded health care systems with some degree of centralised health data collection. For example, the NZ government collects data within a national cancer registry which includes a minimum dataset describing each cancer, alongside mortality, hospital billing information, and data on prescription of pharmaceuticals; similar data exist in some provinces in Canada, and in some states in Australia.

CommNETs is an international collaboration of NET clinicians, researchers and advocates from Australia, NZ and Canada with a mandate to accelerate research in NETs and improve NET care. The need for NET QPIs was identified as a means to monitor and standardise comparisons in order to improve outcomes.

2. Methods

The original process plan used a two-round modified Delphi consensus (RAND/UCLA Appropriateness Method) to select NET-specific QPIs from the QPI literature [25]. However, a literature search returned no relevant results (search strategy Supplementary Material S1). The method was adjusted to include an initial step for generation of candidates for NET QPIs, and is summarised in Figure 1. The first phase (Round 0) aimed to formulate as many measures of NET patient care quality as seen to be relevant. Next, a small group of experts curated the items and made them unambiguous and appropriate for evaluation. Then, Round 1 included a large number of participants from varying disciplines who rated the statements' importance and measurability, in order to identify the top statements. Finally, Round 2 consisted of an expert panel (primarily NET clinicians), who met in person to evaluate the top-ranked statements and provide a final rating.

2.1. Participants

Participants were drawn from the three CommNETs countries (NZ, Canada, Australia), and were multidisciplinary in background, including patients and their advocates (see Figure 1; see Supplementary Material S2).

2.2. Round 0—The Generation of Candidate Statements

Nominal group technique (NGT) is a structured method for idea generation that encourages balanced individual participation; chosen to ensure that the voice of patient advocates and non-clinical disciplines would be heard. NGT was used as previously described [26] and is further summarised in Supplementary Material S3. Participants were allocated into six groups pre-selected to include a range of nationality and multidisciplinary expertise. They received an education session including a background to the project, definitions of QPIs, and the NGT method. Groups generated ideas for NET-specific QPIs for four phases of the NET patient journey. The top five ideas from each phase were taken forward as 'candidates' for assessment in the consensus process. Group membership was changed regularly to encourage new interaction.

2.3. The Conversion of Candidate Statements into Appropriateness Statements

According to the methodology of the modified RAND/UCLA process, "candidates" were converted into statements so that their appropriateness as NET QPIs could be rated. Each appropriateness statement began with the candidate (e.g., *Survival after diagnosis* ...) followed by the phrase " ... *is an important and measurable indicator of NET care quality*". For example, the candidate 'patient reported quality of life' becomes the statement 'patient reported quality of life is an important and measurable indicator of NET care quality.' Some candidates required modification to become 'appropriateness statements'. This curation step (conducted by BL, BW and SP) used the following criteria: candidates with more than one variable or time point were separated into multiple single appropriateness statements; duplicate candidates were discarded; candidates that included multiple concepts were excluded, and candidates with ambiguous statements had additional words added for clarity, with care taken to enhance the intended meaning.

Three factors were repeatedly included in multiple Round 0 candidates; namely site, stage and grade. For example, the candidate "5-year survival by *site, stage and grade*" contains multiple components for ranking, and acknowledges that QPIs vary by site, stage and grade. These three factors were separated and are hereon in referred to as "core indicators." These were presented individually and participants asked whether each was " ... *required to robustly interpret each indicator of NET care quality*". Respondents were, therefore, asked to evaluate the necessity of these core indicators to other indicators, and not their individual importance and measurability.

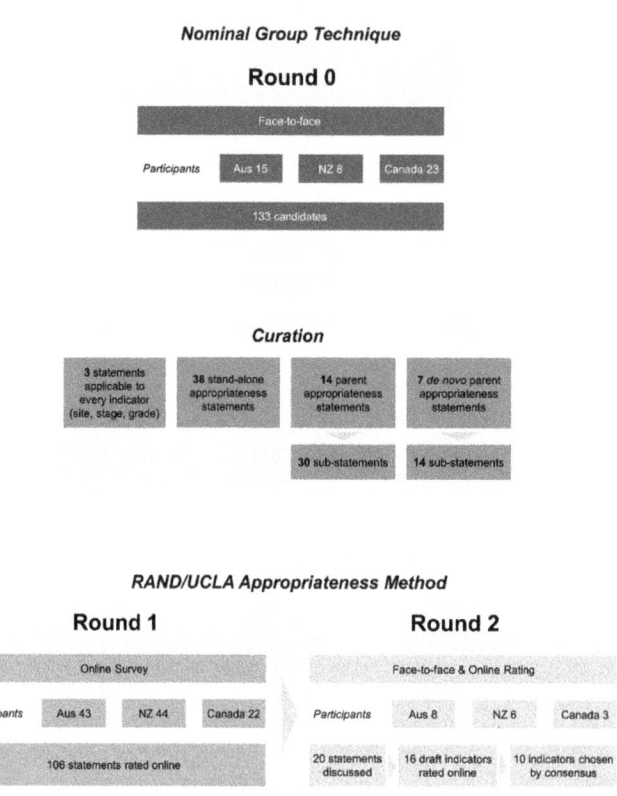

Figure 1. Summary of method. Nominal group technique (NGT) was used to generate 133 "candidates" for neuroendocrine tumour (NET) quality performance indicators (QPIs) (Round 0). These candidates were converted into 106 "appropriateness statements." In Round 1 these statements were evaluated using the RAND/UCLA Appropriateness Method. Participants rated the importance and measurability of each statement as indicators of care quality in an online survey, which led to 20 statements being selected for further discussion. In Round 2, a small group of experts discussed these 20 statements, rejected some, and rated the remainder online, leading to a final list of 10 QPIs.

2.4. Round 1—Online Survey

Survey Monkey® was used to present appropriateness statements and record ratings and feedback. Participants separately rated the *importance* of each statement, and the *measurability* of each statement (see Supplementary Material S4). Participants used a Likert scale to rate each statement from highly inappropriate "1", to uncertain "5", to highly appropriate "9". A weighted average was calculated for positive responses (6–9) using the number of participants and the rating allocated (See Supplementary Material S5). Only responses from participants who completed all fields were included. We arbitrarily determined that statements would be considered important, and measurable, if the positive weighted average was greater than three for both scores.

2.5. Round 2—Modified RAND/UCLA Delphi Consensus Expert Group Ranking

As required by the modified Delphi method, a small expert panel (see Supplementary Material S2, Tables S2 and S3) met to discuss appropriateness statements that had been top ranked in the Round 1 survey, and select a subset of final indicators by consensus. Following the meeting, a rating form was circulated online for rating the draft indicators by the expert group as appropriate, uncertain, or inappropriate. Final NET QPIs were chosen using a consensus threshold of 80%, as utilised in the previous CommNETs Delphi process [27] (see Supplementary Material S6).

3. Results

The number of participants, candidates and appropriateness statements are summarised in Figure 1. Round 0 included 46 multidisciplinary participants (Medical Oncology, Surgery, Endocrinology, Radiation Oncology, Nuclear Medicine, Pathology, Radiology, Research, Pharmacy, Nursing, Patients and their advocates) who produced 133 candidates. Conversion into appropriateness statements required separation of candidates with more than one time point into multiple single statements; duplicates discarded; indicators with multiple concepts excluded, and ambiguity clarified. Statements were organised using a hierarchical structure using appropriateness statements and sub-statements (see Figure 1 and Supplementary Material S3).

The Round 1 survey was sent to 237 people. There were 109 responders, and 71 participants completed all fields in the survey. As some participants sent on the questionnaire to others in their own NET clinical communities, we are unable to calculate an overall response rate. The rating of appropriateness statements in Round 1 showed variable importance (min 1.2, max 3.5) and measurability (min 1.4, max 3.4). Eight statements that were rated as important were not considered measurable. The ratings of the 59 appropriateness statements from Round 1 (after removal of the three core statements, whose importance and measurability were not directly rated) are shown in Figure 2 in order of the weighted average of 'importance' (see Supplementary Material S7 for the corresponding statements). Eight statements (and 13 sub-statements) were rated as both important and measurable (Figure 2). Nine statements (and four sub-statements) were important but not measurable. Forty-two statements (and 17 sub-statements) rated neither important nor measurable.

The small expert group ($n = 17$) met in Round 2 to discuss appropriateness statements indicated by grey dots in Figure 2. This included statements rated both important and measurable in Round 1. The Round 1 ranking methodology could exclude statements because of their wording rather than the value of the concept they described, so several lower-ranked statements were brought forward for 'last chance' discussion by Round 2 participants (as suggested by the RAND/UCLA methodology). The three core statements regarding grade, stage and primary site were also discussed (Table 1). The wording of these statements was sometimes adjusted from the original appropriateness statement in response to discussion. For example three statements related to pathology (Quality of pathology reports; Proportion of histopathology reports presented in a synoptic report; Complete synoptic reporting to College of American Pathologist standards) were combined into a single indicator (Structured pathology report).

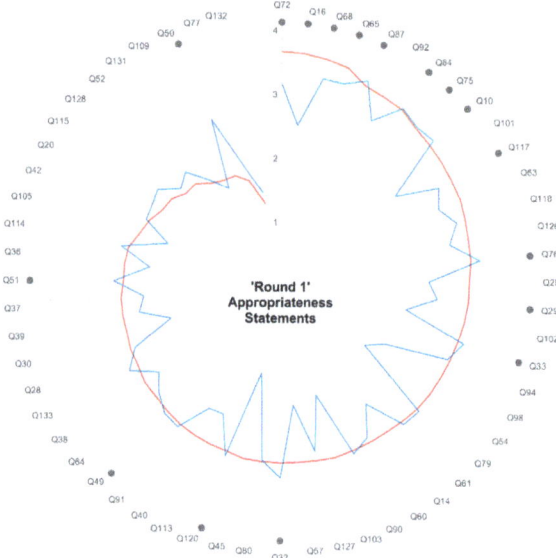

Figure 2. Round 1 ranking of appropriateness statements, ordered by importance. Each radial spoke represents a Round 1 appropriateness statement. Weighted averages for ratings of "Importance" (red line) and "Measurability" (blue line) are presented. Many statements rated as important were not measurable, and a few measurable indicators were not rated as important. Statements taken forward to Round 2 are shown by grey dots, and tended to be both important and measurable (>3 shaded in green). The wording of each statement (e.g., Q72) is shown in Supplementary Material S7.

Table 1. QPI statements assessed in Round 2 and the rationale for further assessment.

Core statements
Grade
Stage
Primary site
Important and measurable statements
Quality of pathology reports
Pathology involvement in MDM review *
MDM review *
Proportion patients with structural imaging
Proportion of patients with functional imaging in staging
Proportion of histopathology reports presented in a synoptic report
Survival after diagnosis
Complete synoptic reporting to College of American Pathologists standards
'Last chance' statements
Proportion of patients receiving systemic treatment
Proportion of patients with surgical consultation for consideration of resection
Proportion of patients who receive surgery with curative intent
Proportion of patients getting resection is an important and measurable indicator of NET care quality
Patient reported quality of life
All cases reported to national registry
Proportion of patients with functional symptom control
Proportion of carcinoid patients who have cardiac imaging
Proportion of NET patients diagnosed with carcinoid heart disease (using echocardiogram)

* Multidisciplinary meeting (MDM) was considered the same as tumour board review.

The final statements ranked online in Round 2 are shown in Figure 3 (*n* = 16). The group agreed that stage, grade and primary site were required to robustly interpret all other indicators, in addition to being quality indicators individually. The presence or absence of metastases was chosen to represent stage, whereas both proliferative index and tumour differentiation were required to represent grade.

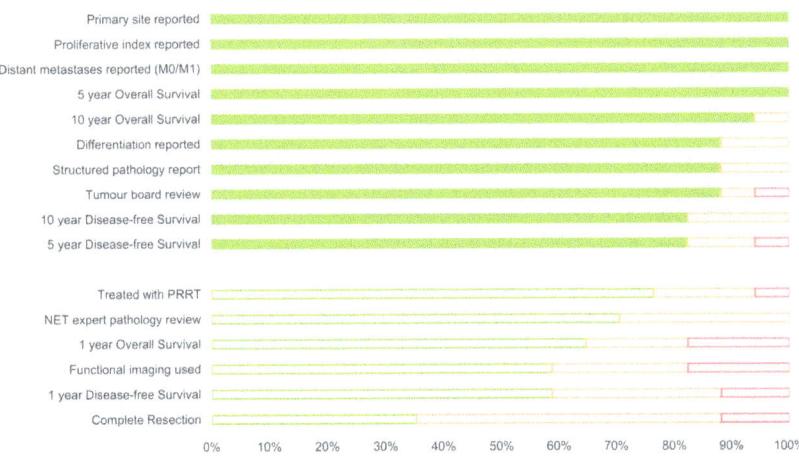

Figure 3. The expert group rated the final Round 2 indicators as appropriate (green), uncertain (orange) or inappropriate (red). The light green shaded area highlights those indicators rated appropriate by more than 80% of the group, thus achieving consensus.

After the face-to-face discussion in Round 2, the 16 draft indicators were rated online. Those indicators rated "appropriate" by at least 80% of the working group were accepted as the final consensus-derived indicators (*n* = 10; Figure 3 and Table 2). Of note, all of the 'last chance' indicators discussed at Round 2 were excluded during this process. The panel noted that proliferative index and differentiation is not required for pheochromocytoma, paraganglioma and medullary thyroid carcinoma.

Table 2. Final consensus-derived NET QPIs.

Primary site reported
Proliferative index reported *
Distant metastases reported (M0/M1)
5-year overall survival
10-year overall survival
Differentiation reported *
Structured pathology report
Tumour board review
5-year disease-free survival
10-year disease-free survival

* this does not currently apply to pheochromocytoma, paraganglioma and medullary thyroid carcinoma.

4. Discussion

In the absence of an evidence base, we used a carefully structured inductive multi-stage process to generate a large set of candidates, and then rate and select QPIs by consensus of experts. The process was deliberately multinational, multidisciplinary, and the patient voice was included at every step. The result is 10 consensus NET QPIs that can be trialled to assess NET care.

The consensus NET QPIs might appear generic at first glance, but review of discussion transcripts and notes suggests that the QPIs capture aspects of diagnosis and care that are inherent to NET outcome. Three of the 10 QPIs are pathology-focused, acknowledging the heterogeneity and variable biology of NETs. 'Proliferative index reported' and 'Differentiation reported' form the basis of grade and determine outcome in most NETs, and 'Structured pathology report' acknowledges the need for consistent reporting of these fundamental attributes. NET rarity, heterogeneity and the multidisciplinary nature of NET care is acknowledged in 'Tumour board review'. The inclusion of 'Primary site reported' recognises that different clinical behaviour is observed from different NET primary sites, but also the variable quality of staging of NETs in the metastatic setting, and variable access to NET-specific imaging such as Ga68-DOTA-tate PET CT. In the same way, 'Distant metastases reported' acknowledges both the requirement for and quality of radiological staging in most NETs. Finally, the time points of the four survival QPIs were skewed to match the natural history of NETs, recognising the predominantly favourable disease course with 5- and 10-year measures rather than the shorter time frames used in other cancer types.

The rigorous assessment of measurability excluded many potentially important QPIs, leading to limitations in the consensus NET QPIs. There are no QPIs that address the time from first symptom to diagnosis, treatment provision, or follow-up after resection. In these situations, reliable and measurable QPIs could not be agreed. There are no indicators with highly granular outcomes specific to NETs, such as echocardiographic assessment of carcinoid heart disease and there are no outcome measures specific to high grade NETs (e.g., 1-year overall survival). In addition, no indicators relating to the functional aspects of NETs were selected as a QPI. The relevant statements were not considered to be of sufficient applicability to NETs as a whole, although it was recognised that they could be valuable in specific settings and NET subtypes. The functional imaging QPI was rated as appropriate by 60% of the final Round 2 group and, therefore, did not meet the criteria for inclusion as a consensus derived QPI. This potentially reflects both the heterogeneity of NETs (functional imaging is not required for care of some NETs) and access to functional imaging in different health systems. Not all patients with NETs require functional imaging, and the utility of radiotracers varies with grade of NET and over time within individuals with NETs. As a QPI, functional imaging would measure how often functional imaging is used, and whether it is available and utilised in the appropriate setting (e.g., detection of occult primary, pre-operative staging, and for selection of patients for peptide receptor radionuclide therapy). As access to functional imaging becomes more universal, the value of a functional imaging QPI is likely to increase.

The outcome QPIs describe long time frames that are appropriate for the biological behaviour of NETs, but will make actionability difficult due to the delay in seeing the impact of any intervention. This may restrict 10-year survival to use in retrospective comparison, rather than prospective monitoring of ongoing care. Multiple measures of survival were identified as candidates in Round 0 (including overall survival, disease-free survival, progression free survival and disease control rate) but only overall survival and disease-free survival were included in the final 10 indicators. Overall survival is the most easily measured outcome measure, using mortality data, and is important for all NETs. Progression free survival, disease-free survival and disease control rate are less easily measured using routinely collected data in most jurisdictions. The inclusion of disease-free survival as a QPI reflects its importance in measuring outcome in NET patients receiving curative treatment.

The modified RAND/UCLA Delphi method used for NET QPI development is essentially qualitative, and care is needed to avoid introducing bias. For example, the project had been planned to review existing evidence-based indicators from the literature, but we generated draft indicators de novo which is inferior to selection from factors known to be associated with survival (or meaningful patient reported outcomes). Bias could be introduced at each phase of NET QPI development. The statements generated in Round 0 using NGT might reflect the beliefs of participants; careful use of multidisciplinary members, assigned group membership and a method that encouraged participation was used to ameliorate this. The Round 1 questionnaire was moderately arduous (62 statements, with sub-statements in check boxes), which might have introduced bias by retrieving opinions from only the most engaged participants. Participants in Round 2 were able to 'bring forward' lower ranked statements for further discussion (as required by the RAND/UCLA method) to address missing parts of the patient journey, or highly aspirational indicators that might not have fared well in Round 1 online assessment. This could also introduce bias, but interestingly, none of these added statements were valued highly enough in Round 2 to make it to the final consensus list. This implies validity for the Round 1 ranking process; only indicators that had been ranked as important AND measurable in Round 1 were finally accepted as the consensus QPIs after Round 2.

It is also interesting to consider the level of expertise indirectly recommended by each consensus NET QPI, and the point on a continuum from generalist through to 'NET-specific expert' needed to achieve each QPI. To explain, the Round 2 expert group assessed several statements that required a very high level of NET expert care: such as review in a "NET-specific" tumour board, review by a "NET expert" pathologist, the use of functional imaging; and availability of radionuclide therapy. These four statements did not reach the consensus threshold and were rejected; for example, review by any type of tumour board was deemed acceptable, thus advocating tertiary- but not quaternary-level review. This was thought to facilitate a reasonable standard of care across the three CommNETs countries at this point in time, and might help translation of the QPIs to other countries outside CommNETs. Arguably, these more aspirational indicators should be monitored and assessed for inclusion in future NET QPI sets if the provision of clinical care catches up with the aspirations of the providers.

These QPIs were developed with the aim of measuring care quality across health care systems, but can also provide a guide to individual physicians in their care of people with NETs, particularly the non-outcome based QPIs. For example, at diagnosis, has the primary site been identified and is staging complete? Are grade and pathological differentiation reported in a structured pathology report? If not, imaging and formal pathological review should be requested, with additional imaging and pathological assessment undertaken as required to obtain primary site, stage and grade. Discussion at a multidisciplinary team meeting or tumour board is recommended, and may facilitate obtaining this key information. In this way, the consensus NET QPIs will help improve care of people with NETs and increase the comfort of clinicians caring for people with NETs at an individual level. The next stage of this project will be to measure performance on these QPIs and feed back to providers; this feedback is expected to change clinician behavior by providing both a tacit message of what is required for good care, and by showing each organisation where they are under-performing.

A number of organisations have published management guidelines for NETs that cover aspects of care including diagnosis, imaging, surgical and systemic therapies, and follow up for NETs originating in different anatomical locations [28–34]. As noted above, the heterogeneity seen in NETs is one of the challenging features in designing QPIs, and similarly there are multiple guidelines for each primary site. The proposed QPIs can be conceptualized as a highly measurable and concise subset of these many guidelines. The molecular make up of NETs and how this impacts on treatment response is an area of active research, and as the understanding of molecular subtypes evolves these will become potential candidate indicators in the future.

This project will now move to trialing of the consensus NET QPIs, initially by application to retrospective registry data. The aim is to understand associations between the NET QPIs that describe diagnosis and investigation, with those that describe outcome. The role of the NET QPIs for international comparison will be assessed. The selection of QPIs is a dynamic process and should be kept under regular review and adapted to changes according to emerging evidence and clinical practice. Considered debate will be undertaken to decide how QPIs are reported to stakeholders.

5. Conclusions

This CommNETs project has developed and refined a small set of consensus NET QPIs. These NET QPIs will now be trialed as a method to monitor and improve care for people with NETs and to facilitate international comparison.

Supplementary Materials: The following are available online at http://www.mdpi.com/2077-0383/8/9/1455/s1: Material S1: Literature Search, Material S2: Participants, Material S3: 'Round 0' methodology, Material S4: 'Round

1' Online Survey, Material S5: Weighted score, Material S6: Round 2—modified RAND/UCLA Delphi Consensus expert group ranking, Material S7: Round 1 results index.

Author Contributions: Conceptualization, B.L., S.P., S.S., E.S., D.W., and M.M.; methodology B.L., B.W. and S.P.; formal analysis, B.W., B.L., S.P., E.S., S.S., K.P., G.K., W.M., D.W., N.P., S.C., V.G., J.K., N.K., M.M., K.W., T.A., G.M-R., D.L. and T.P.; investigation, B.W., B.L., S.P., E.S., S.S., K.P., G.K., W.M., D.W., N.P., S.C., V.G., J.K., N.K., M.M., K.W., T.A., G.M-R., D.L. and T.P.; resources, B.L., S.P., B.W. and K.P.; data curation, B.L., S.P., B.W. and K.P.; writing—original draft preparation, B.L., B.W. and S.P.; writing—review and editing, B.W., B.L., S.P., E.S., S.S., K.P., G.K., W.M., D.W., N.P., S.C., V.G., J.K., N.K., M.M., K.W., T.A., G.M-R., D.L. and T.P.; visualization, B.W. and B.L.; project administration, B.W., K.P. and B.L.; funding acquisition, B.L.

Funding: B.W. is a member of the NETwork! Research group in New Zealand. He was funded to assist this project by the Ministry of Health, New Zealand Government, Wellington, New Zealand.

Acknowledgments: Additional CommNETs collaborators who participated in the initial development of candidate indicators; Matthew Anaka, University of Toronto, Toronto, Canada; Timothy Asmis, Ottawa Hospital Cancer Centre, Ottawa, Canada; Jamil Asselah, McGill University Health Centre, Montreal, Canada; Jonathan Boekhoud, Cancer Care Ontario, Toronto, Canada; Cynthia Card, University of Calgary, Calgary, Canada; Richard Carroll, Capital & Coast DHB Endocrine Service, Wellington, New Zealand; Gabrielle Cehic, The Queen Elizabeth Hospital, Woodville, Australia; A/Prof Prosanto Chaudhury, McGill University Health Centre, Montreal, Canada; Nadia Corsini, University of South Australia, Adelaide, Australia; Marianne Elston, Waikato Hospital, Hamilton, New Zealand; Rachel Goodwin, Ottawa Hospital Cancer Centre, Ottawa, Canada; Ms Alana Gould, Capital & Coast DHB Endocrine Service, Wellington, New Zealand; A/Prof Daryl Gray, London Health Sciences Centre, London, Canada; Aimee Hayes, Royal North Shore Hospital, Sydney, Australia; Dev Kevat, Monash Health, Melbourne, Australia; David Laidley, Western University, London, Canada; Prof Calvin Law, Sunnybrook Health Science Centre, Toronto, Canada; Ms Simone Leyden, Unicorn Foundation, Melbourne, Australia; Amanda Love, Royal Brisbane and Women's Hospital, Brisbane, Australia; Mr Enrico Mandarino, CNETs Canada, Cornwall, Canada; Celia Marginean, Ottawa Hospital, Ottawa, Canada; Lucy Modahl, Auckland Radiology Group, Auckland, New Zealand; Mrs Jan Mumford, AGITG Consumer Advisory Panel Chair, Australia; Sten Myrehaug, Odette Cancer Centre, Toronto, Canada; A/Prof Chris O'Callaghan, Canadian Cancer Trials Group, Kingston, Canada; Dainik Patel, Lyell McEwin Hospital, Adelaide, Australia; David Ransom, Fiona Stanley Hospital, Murdoch, Australia; A/Prof Paul Roach, Royal North Shore Hospital, Sydney, Australia; A/Prof Andrew Strickland, Monash Health, Melbourne, Australia; Ms Alia Thawer, Odette Cancer Centre, Toronto, Canada; Michael Vickers, Ottawa Hospital Cancer Centre, Ottawa, Canada; Marguerite Wieler, University of Alberta, Edmonton, Canada; Bin Xu, Sunnybrook Health Sciences Centre, Toronto, Canada; Radhika Yelamanchili, Walker Family Cancer Centre, Niagara Region, Canada; and all those CommNETs collaborators who participated in the Round 1 online survey.

Conflicts of Interest: The authors declare no relevant conflict of interest. The funders had no role in the design of the study; in the collection, analyses, or interpretation of data; in the writing of the manuscript; or in the decision to publish the results.

References

1. New Zealand Ministry of Health. *Bowel Cancer Quality Performance Indicators: Descriptions*; Ministry of Health: Wellington, New Zealand, 2019.
2. Cancer Australia. National Cancer Control Indicators (NCCI). Available online: https://ncci.canceraustralia.gov.au (accessed on 20 June 2019).
3. New Zealand Ministry of Health Cancer Services. Review of the National Tumour Standards. Available online: https://www.health.govt.nz/our-work/diseases-and-conditions/national-cancer-programme/cancer-initiatives/review-national-tumour-standards (accessed on 20 June 2019).
4. Cancer Quality Council of Ontario. Cancer System Quality Index (CSQI). Available online: https://www.csqi.on.ca/indicators (accessed on 20 June 2019).
5. The Scottish Government. Healthcare and Healthcare Improvement—National Cancer Quality Programme. Available online: https://www.sehd.scot.nhs.uk/mels/CEL2012_06.pdf (accessed on 20 June 2019).
6. National Quality Forum. NQF Endorses Cancer Measures. Available online: https://www.qualityforum.org/News_And_Resources/Press_Releases/2012/NQF_Endorses_Cancer_Measures.aspx (accessed on 20 June 2019).
7. Stordeur, S.; Vrijens, F.; Beirens, K.; Vlayen, J.; Devriese, S.; Van Eycken, E. *Quality Indicators in Oncology: Breast Cancer. Good Clinical Practice (GCP)*; Belgian Health Care Knowledge Centre (KCE): Brussels, Belgium, 2010.
8. Walpole, E.T.; Theile, D.E.; Philpot, S.; Youl, P.H. Development and Implementation of a Cancer Quality Index in Queensland, Australia: A Tool for Monitoring Cancer Care. *J. Oncol. Pract.* **2019**, *15*, e636–e643. [CrossRef] [PubMed]

9. Scottish Cancer Taskforce and National Cancer Quality Steering Group. Lung Cancer Clinical Quality Performance Indicators. Available online: http://www.healthcareimprovementscotland.org/our_work/cancer_care_improvement/cancer_qpis/quality_performance_indicators.aspx (accessed on 20 Jun 2019).
10. Biganzoli, L.; Marotti, L.; Hart, C.D.; Cataliotti, L.; Cutuli, B.; Kuhn, T.; Mansel, R.E.; Ponti, A.; Poortmans, P.; Regitnig, P.; et al. Quality indicators in breast cancer care: An update from the EUSOMA working group. *Eur. J. Cancer* **2017**, *86*, 59–81. [CrossRef] [PubMed]
11. Watanabe, T.; Mikami, M.; Katabuchi, H.; Kato, S.; Kaneuchi, M.; Takahashi, M.; Nakai, H.; Nagase, S.; Niikura, H.; Mandai, M.; et al. Quality indicators for cervical cancer care in Japan. *J. Gynecol. Oncol.* **2018**, *29*, e83. [CrossRef] [PubMed]
12. Maharaj, A.D.; Ioannou, L.; Croagh, D.; Zalcberg, J.; Neale, R.E.; Goldstein, D.; Merrett, N.; Kench, J.G.; White, K.; Pilgrim, C.H.C.; et al. Monitoring quality of care for patients with pancreatic cancer: A modified Delphi consensus. *HPB (Oxford)* **2019**, *21*, 444–455. [CrossRef] [PubMed]
13. New Zealand Ministry of Health. Bowel Cancer Quality Performance Indicator Specifications. Available online: https://www.health.govt.nz/publication/bowel-cancer-quality-performance-indicator-specifications (accessed on 29 July 2019).
14. Gagliardi, A.R.; Simunovic, M.; Langer, B.; Stern, H.; Brown, A.D. Development of quality indicators for colorectal cancer surgery, using a 3-step modified Delphi approach. *Can. J. Surg.* **2005**, *48*, 441–452. [PubMed]
15. Di Valentin, T.; Biagi, J.; Bourque, S.; Butt, R.; Champion, P.; Chaput, V.; Colwell, B.; Cripps, C.; Dorreen, M.; Edwards, S.; et al. Eastern Canadian Colorectal Cancer Consensus Conference: Standards of care for the treatment of patients with rectal, pancreatic, and gastrointestinal stromal tumours and pancreatic neuroendocrine tumours. *Curr. Oncol.* **2013**, *20*, e455–e464. [CrossRef] [PubMed]
16. Khare, S.R.; Batist, G.; Bartlett, G. Identification of performance indicators across a network of clinical cancer programs. *Curr. Oncol.* **2016**, *23*, 81–90. [CrossRef]
17. Turner, N.H.; Wong, H.L.; Field, K.; Wong, R.; Shapiro, J.; Yip, D.; Nott, L.; Tie, J.; Kosmider, S.; Tran, B.; et al. Novel quality indicators for metastatic colorectal cancer management identify significant variations in these measures across treatment centers in Australia. *Asia Pac. J. Clin. Oncol.* **2015**, *11*, 262–271. [CrossRef]
18. Man, D.; Wu, J.; Shen, Z.; Zhu, X. Prognosis of patients with neuroendocrine tumor: A SEER database analysis. *Cancer Manag. Res.* **2018**, *10*, 5629–5638. [CrossRef]
19. Dasari, A.; Shen, C.; Halperin, D.; Zhao, B.; Zhou, S.; Xu, Y.; Shih, T.; Yao, J.C. Trends in the Incidence, Prevalence, and Survival Outcomes in Patients With Neuroendocrine Tumors in the United States. *JAMA Oncol.* **2017**, *3*, 1335–1342. [CrossRef]
20. Hallet, J.; Law, C.H.; Cukier, M.; Saskin, R.; Liu, N.; Singh, S. Exploring the rising incidence of neuroendocrine tumors: A population-based analysis of epidemiology, metastatic presentation, and outcomes. *Cancer* **2015**, *121*, 589–597. [CrossRef] [PubMed]
21. Lawrence, B.; Gustafsson, B.I.; Chan, A.; Svejda, B.; Kidd, M.; Modlin, I.M. The epidemiology of gastroenteropancreatic neuroendocrine tumors. *Endocrinol. Metab. Clin. N. Am.* **2011**, *40*, 1–18. [CrossRef] [PubMed]
22. Perez, E.A.; Koniaris, L.G.; Snell, S.E.; Gutierrez, J.C.; Sumner, W.E., III; Lee, D.J.; Hodgson, N.C.; Livingstone, A.S.; Franceschi, D. 7201 carcinoids: Increasing incidence overall and disproportionate mortality in the elderly. *World J. Surg.* **2007**, *31*, 1022–1030. [CrossRef] [PubMed]
23. Yao, J.C.; Hassan, M.; Phan, A.; Dagohoy, C.; Leary, C.; Mares, J.E.; Abdalla, E.K.; Fleming, J.B.; Vauthey, J.N.; Rashid, A.; et al. One hundred years after "carcinoid": Epidemiology of and prognostic factors for neuroendocrine tumors in 35,825 cases in the United States. *J. Clin. Oncol.* **2008**, *26*, 3063–3072. [CrossRef] [PubMed]
24. Hallet, J.; Coburn, N.G.; Singh, S.; Beyfuss, K.; Koujanian, S.; Liu, N.; Law, C.H.L. Access to care and outcomes for neuroendocrine tumours: Does socioeconomic status matter? *Curr. Oncol.* **2018**, *25*, e356–e364. [CrossRef] [PubMed]
25. Fitch, K.; Bernstein, S.J.; Aguilar, M.D.; Burnand, B.; LaCalle, J.R. *The RAND/UCLA Appropriateness Method User's Manual*; RAND Corporation: Santa Monica, CA, USA, 2001.
26. American Society for Quality. About Nominal Group Technique. Available online: https://asq.org/quality-resources/nominal-group-technique (accessed on 23 May 2019).

27. Segelov, E.; Chan, D.; Lawrence, B.; Pavlakis, N.; Kennecke, H.F.; Jackson, C.; Law, C.; Singh, S. Identifying and Prioritizing Gaps in Neuroendocrine Tumor Research: A Modified Delphi Process With Patients and Health Care Providers to Set the Research Action Plan for the Newly Formed Commonwealth Neuroendocrine Tumor Collaboration. *J. Glob. Oncol.* **2017**, *3*, 380–388. [CrossRef] [PubMed]
28. Singh, S.; Moody, L.; Chan, D.L.; Metz, D.C.; Strosberg, J.; Asmis, T.; Bailey, D.L.; Bergsland, E.; Brendtro, K.; Carroll, R.; et al. Follow-up Recommendations for Completely Resected Gastroenteropancreatic Neuroendocrine Tumors. *JAMA Oncol.* **2018**, *4*, 1597–1604. [CrossRef] [PubMed]
29. Delle Fave, G.; O'Toole, D.; Sundin, A.; Taal, B.; Ferolla, P.; Ramage, J.K.; Ferone, D.; Ito, T.; Weber, W.; Zheng-Pei, Z.; et al. ENETS Consensus Guidelines Update for Gastroduodenal Neuroendocrine Neoplasms. *Neuroendocrinology* **2016**, *103*, 119–124. [CrossRef] [PubMed]
30. Pavel, M.; O'Toole, D.; Costa, F.; Capdevila, J.; Gross, D.; Kianmanesh, R.; Krenning, E.; Knigge, U.; Salazar, R.; Pape, U.F.; et al. ENETS Consensus Guidelines Update for the Management of Distant Metastatic Disease of Intestinal, Pancreatic, Bronchial Neuroendocrine Neoplasms (NEN) and NEN of Unknown Primary Site. *Neuroendocrinology* **2016**, *103*, 172–185. [CrossRef]
31. Strosberg, J.R.; Halfdanarson, T.R.; Bellizzi, A.M.; Chan, J.A.; Dillon, J.S.; Heaney, A.P.; Kunz, P.L.; O'Dorisio, T.M.; Salem, R.; Segelov, E.; et al. The North American Neuroendocrine Tumor Society Consensus Guidelines for Surveillance and Medical Management of Midgut Neuroendocrine Tumors. *Pancreas* **2017**, *46*, 707–714. [CrossRef]
32. Howe, J.R.; Cardona, K.; Fraker, D.L.; Kebebew, E.; Untch, B.R.; Wang, Y.Z.; Law, C.H.; Liu, E.H.; Kim, M.K.; Menda, Y.; et al. The Surgical Management of Small Bowel Neuroendocrine Tumors: Consensus Guidelines of the North American Neuroendocrine Tumor Society. *Pancreas* **2017**, *46*, 715–731. [CrossRef] [PubMed]
33. Perren, A.; Couvelard, A.; Scoazec, J.Y.; Costa, F.; Borbath, I.; Delle Fave, G.; Gorbounova, V.; Gross, D.; Grossma, A.; Jense, R.T.; et al. ENETS Consensus Guidelines for the Standards of Care in Neuroendocrine Tumors: Pathology: Diagnosis and Prognostic Stratification. *Neuroendocrinology* **2017**, *105*, 196–200. [CrossRef] [PubMed]
34. Kunz, P.L.; Reidy-Lagunes, D.; Anthony, L.B.; Bertino, E.M.; Brendtro, K.; Chan, J.A.; Chen, H.; Jensen, R.T.; Kim, M.K.; Klimstra, D.S.; et al. Consensus guidelines for the management and treatment of neuroendocrine tumors. *Pancreas* **2013**, *42*, 557–577. [CrossRef] [PubMed]

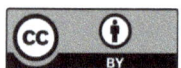

© 2019 by the authors. Licensee MDPI, Basel, Switzerland. This article is an open access article distributed under the terms and conditions of the Creative Commons Attribution (CC BY) license (http://creativecommons.org/licenses/by/4.0/).

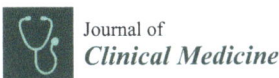

Article

Safety and Activity of Metronomic Temozolomide in Second-Line Treatment of Advanced Neuroendocrine Neoplasms

Salvatore Tafuto [1,2,†], Claudia von Arx [1,2,3,†], Monica Capozzi [1,2,*], Fabiana Tatangelo [2,4], Manuela Mura [2,3], Roberta Modica [2,5], Maria Luisa Barretta [2,6], Antonella Di Sarno [2,7], Maria Lina Tornesello [2,8], Annamaria Colao [2,5] and Alessandro Ottaiano [1,2]

1. Department of Abdominal Oncology, Istituto Nazionale Tumori, IRCCS-Fondazione "G. Pascale", 80131 Naples, Italy
2. ENETs (European NeuroEndocrine Tumors Society), Center of Excellence of Naples, 80131 Naples, Italy
3. Department of Surgery and Cancer, Imperial College London, London W12 0HS, UK
4. Department of Pathology, Istituto Nazionale Tumori, IRCCS-Fondazione "G. Pascale", 80131 Naples, Italy
5. Department of Clinical Medicine and Surgery, Federico II University, 80131 Naples, Italy
6. UOC of Radiology, Istituto Nazionale Tumori, IRCCS-Fondazione "G. Pascale", 80131 Naples, Italy
7. UOC of Oncology, A.O. dei Colli, Monaldi Unit, 80131 Naples, Italy
8. Molecular Biology and Viral Oncology Unit, Istituto Nazionale Tumori IRCCS "Fondazione G. Pascale", 80131 Naples, Italy
* Correspondence: monicacapozzi@virgilio.it; Tel.: +39-0815-903680
† These authors contributed equally to this work.

Received: 11 July 2019; Accepted: 12 August 2019; Published: 15 August 2019

Abstract: Background. Platinum-based chemotherapy is the mainstay of front-line treatment of patients affected by pluri-metastatic intermediate/high grade NeuroEndocrine Neoplasms (NENs). However, there are no standard second-line treatments at disease progression. Previous clinical experiences have evidenced that temozolomide (TMZ), an oral analog of dacarbazine, is active against NENs at standard doses of 150 to 200 mg/mq per day on days 1 to 5 of a 28-day cycle, even if a significant treatment-related toxicity is reported. Methods. Metastatic NENs patients were treated at the ENETS (European NeuroEndocrine Tumor Society) center of excellence of Naples (Italy), from 2014 to 2017 with a second-line alternative metronomic schedule of TMZ, 75 mg/m^2 *per os* "one week on/one week off". Toxicity was graded with NCI-CTC criteria v4.0; objective responses with RECIST v1.1 and performance status (PS) according to ECOG. Results. Twenty-six consecutive patients were treated. Median age was 65.5 years. The predominant primary organs were pancreas and lung. Grading was G2 in 11 patients, G3 in 15. More than half of patients had a PS 2 (15 vs. 11 with PS 1). The median time-on-temozolomide therapy was 12.2 months (95% CI: 11.4–19.6). No G3/G4 toxicities were registered. Complete response was obtained in 1 patient, partial response in 4, stable disease in 19 (disease control rate: 92.3%), and progressive disease in 2. The median overall survival from TMZ start was 28.3 months. PS improved in 73% of patients. Conclusions. Metronomic TMZ is a suitable treatment for G2 and G3 NENs particularly in PS 2 patients. Prospective and larger trials are needed to confirm these results.

Keywords: neuroendocrine neoplasms; chemotherapy; temozolomide; metronomic treatment; second-line

1. Introduction

NeuroEndocrine Neoplasms (NENs) are a group of tumors arising from the neuroendocrine cell compartment present in different tissues [1,2]. Their management is complex and depends on tumor grading, differentiation, proliferation index and presence of specific syndromes and/or metastases [3]. The front-line treatment of pluri-metastatic intermediate/high grade NENs is based on systemic platinum-based chemotherapies [4,5]. However, when the disease progresses, there is a lack of evidence for standard second-line treatments.

Temozolomide (TMZ) is an orally active alkylating agent analogue of the dacarbazine. In monotherapy and at the standard doses of 150–200 mg/m^2 once daily for 5 every 28 days, TMZ showed to be active in pre-treated patients affected by NENs with response rates (RR) of 14% in patient with G1/G2 NENs [6] and a disease control rate (DCR) of 38% in G3 NeuroEndocrine Carcinomas (NECs) [7]. In association with other drugs, namely capecitabine, everolimus, bevacizumab and octreotide, and thalidomide the RR ranges between 17–70% [8–16]. The large part of these studies is small (<25 patients) and/or retrospective because of the low incidence of the disease. The most frequent reported all-grade toxicities of TMZ single-agent or combined with other drugs are anemia, leucopenia, thrombocytopenia, hand-foot syndrome and gastrointestinal. However, a discontinuation rate of TMZ up to 55% is reported [16], and in association with everolimus, the treatment with TMZ has been precautionary administrated for a maximum of 6 months in order to reduce toxicity [13].

The use a metronomic schedule of TMZ represents a possible way to reduce toxicity. Metronomic TMZ (mTMZ) consists on lower daily doses with greater frequency of administration. The main biological effects reside on anti-angiogenic activity [17–19] and immune-modulation leading to improvement of dendritic cells function [20] and selective depletion of CD4$^+$CD25$^+$Foxp3$^+$ regulatory T cells (Tregs), which are potent immunosuppressive cells within the tumor microenvironment [21–24].

There are no studies in literature evaluating the activity and safety of mTMZ in advanced pre-treated intermediate/high grade NENs. In this study, we evaluated the efficacy of mTMZ in a consecutive series of 26 NENs patients treated at the ENETS (European NeuroEndocrine Tumor Society) center of Naples.

2. Experimental Section

2.1. Patients, Treatment and Disease Characteristics

This was a retrospective study approved by the Scientific Directorate (among criteria: Reliable and verifiable source of data, consecutiveness of the cases to reduce biases, adequate follow-up, monocentric radiologic evaluations) of the National Cancer Institute of Naples and conducted at the ENETS Center of Excellence in Naples (Italy). The ENETS center of Naples internal database collects data about NENs' patients from three different institutions; it was utilized to identify consecutive cases of patients with advanced G2-G3 NENs (Naples, Italy), progressed after a first-line systemic therapy and treated with second-line mTMZ therapy between 2014 and 2017. All patients had progressive and measurable metastatic disease with an Eastern Cooperative Oncology Group Performance Status (ECOG PS) from 0 to 2 and life expectancy greater than three months. Adequate hematological, renal, and hepatic function with laboratory values demonstrating WBC ≥3000/mm^3, platelet count ≥100,000/mm^3, hemoglobin >8.0 g/dL, ALT and AST≤ to 3.5 times the upper limit of normal, creatinine ≤1.6 mg/dL, and total bilirubin ≤2.0 mg/dL were also required. Patients were excluded in case of active systemic infections, coagulation disorders or decompensated chronic illnesses. Following the procedures of our Institute, retrospective studies are submitted only to the approval of Scientific Directorate and do not require ethical approval.

The treatment schedule consisted on oral administration of "one week on/one week off" TMZ at 75 mg/m^2 until unacceptable toxicity or progression. The drug was taken on an empty stomach (1 h before or 2 h after eating), with a full glass of water. Written informed consent was obtained before prescribing and starting therapy. Data about patients and disease characteristics (age, gender, PS, comorbidities, stage), histology (primary tumor site and size, Ki67 status), previous treatments (surgery and/or systemic treatments) were shown in Table 1. The median age was 65.5 years (range: 32–88 years) and the genders were equally represented (13 patients were male and 13 patients were female). Fifteen patients (58%) had an ECOG PS of 2 before starting the second line treatment, while 11 patients (42%) presented with a PS equal to 1. No patient had a PS of 0. Grading is a fundamental characteristic to drive therapeutic choices, G2 NENs were 42% and G3 58%. Among the G3 NENs, 10 out of 15 (67%) had a Ki67 between 20% and 55%. The predominant primary sites were pancreas and lung, whereas the predominant site of metastasis was the liver followed by loco-regional nodes and bone. In half of the patients, metastases were present in a single site, and the liver was the only involved site in the 81% of patients. In contrast, 8 patients (31%) had two different sites of metastasis, and in 5 patients (19%) the sites of metastasis were equal or more than three. The majority of patients (54%) was previously treated with chemotherapy, whereas 31% received Somato Statin Analogues (SSAs) as first line treatment, and 15% received other treatments including immunotherapy or targeted/biologic therapies. Of the 14 patients who received first line chemotherapy, 12 received platinum-based treatments and two non-platinum chemotherapy regimens. In addition, among the chemo-treated patients, 10 (71%) had a G3 NEN but 4 (29%) had a G2 NEN. In the latter patients, the choice to administer chemotherapy was based on the primary site of the NENs and/or on the Ki67: two atypical carcinoids with a Ki67 ≥ 15%, one intracranial neuroendocrine tumor and one NEN of unknown primary origin with a Ki67 of 18%. Of the 8 patients who received SSAs, half received octreotide and half lanreotide.

Table 1. Characteristics of patients and disease.

Characteristics	No.
Age, years	
Median	65
Range	32–88
Gender	
Male	13
Female	13
Grading	
G1	0
G2	11
G3 *	15
KI-67 level	
3–20	11
20–55	10
>55	5
Performance Status	
0	0
1	11
2	15
Site of primary tumor	
Pancreas	5
Lung	5
Stomach	3
Miscellanea	
Head and Neck	2
Small bowel	3
Rectum	1
Gallbladder	1
Cutaneous	1
Unknown Primary Origin	5
No. of involved metastatic sites	
1	13
2	8
≥3	5
Previous treatments	
Platinum-based treatments	12
Chemotherapy non-platinum based	2
Somatostatin analogues	8
Clinical trials drugs	4

* 3 Large Cell NECs were included, small-cell types were not included.

2.2. Activity, Toxicity and Clinical Benefit Evaluations

Tumor assessment was performed every three months through Computed Tomography (CT) scans. Responses to treatment were defined according to RECIST 1.1 (Response Evaluation Criteria in Solid Tumors) [20]. Complete response (CR) was defined as the disappearance of all lesions, and partial response (PR) as a decrease of 30% or more in the sum of the longest diameters. Progressive disease (PD) was defined as either the appearance of new lesions or an increase of 20% or more compared with the minimum sum of longest diameters recorded since the start of treatment. Stable disease (SD) was defined when the sum increased by <20% or decreased by <30% and no new lesions appeared. The objective response rate (ORR) was the sum of CRs + PRs. The disease control rate (DCR) was the sum of CRs + PRs + SDs.

Adverse events were graded according to the National Cancer Institute Common Terminology Criteria for Adverse Events (NCI-CTCAE version 4) [25]. Physical examination, complete blood counts and blood chemical tests were carried out once a week until the end of the second month and once every 2 weeks thereafter. For each adverse event, the maximum grade per patient was reported. If a patient experienced a toxic effect of any grade on multiple occasions, the event was counted only once. Patients' toxicities attributable to prior first-line treatment must have recovered to a grade 1 or less (except for alopecia) before starting mTMZ. No grade 3 or 4 toxicities were observed. Grade 2 non-hematologic toxicities were managed by cessation of the drug until resolution to grade 1 and then resuming treatment without a dose reduction. Neither treatment delays nor reductions were applied in case of hematologic grade 1 or 2 or non-hematologic grade 1 toxicities.

The clinical benefit was defined as an improvement of the ECOG PS assessed before starting mTMZ, at 3 and 6 months.

2.3. Time-to-Outcome Analysis and Statistical Methods

Data are predominantly descriptive. Progression free survival (PFS) was calculated as the time elapsed from the date of mTMZ initiation to the date of disease progression or death for any cause (whichever occurred first). Patients who were alive with no disease progression were censored at the date of last visit. Overall Survival (OS) was defined as the time from the start of mTMZ administration to the date of death for any cause. Patients who were alive were censored at the date of data analysis. The median PFS (mPFS) and the median OS (mOS) curves were depicted using the Kaplan-Meier method. Exploratory subgroup analyses were done by Log-rank test.

3. Results

Efficacy and Safety

From 2014 to 2017, twenty-six consecutive patients with advanced G2-G3 NENs in progression after a first line chemotherapy were treated with second-line mTMZ. Characteristics of patients and their disease have been described in the Experimental Section. At last follow-up (median follow-up from mTMZ start: 29 months), 16 (62%) patients were alive, and 8 (31%) were still on treatment with mTMZ. All patients were evaluable for response. The objective response rate (ORR) to second-line mTMZ was 19%, with one complete response (CR) and four partial responses (PR). An additional 73% of patients achieved stable disease (SD) as best response (Table 2 and Figure 1a).

Table 2. Efficacy estimates of second-line mTMZ.

Response to Therapy	No. (%)
Complete Response	1 (3.8)
Partial Response	4 (15.4)
Stable Disease	19 (73.1)
Progressive Disease	2 (7.6)
Median PFS (18 events)	9.0 months
Median OS (10 events)	28.3 months

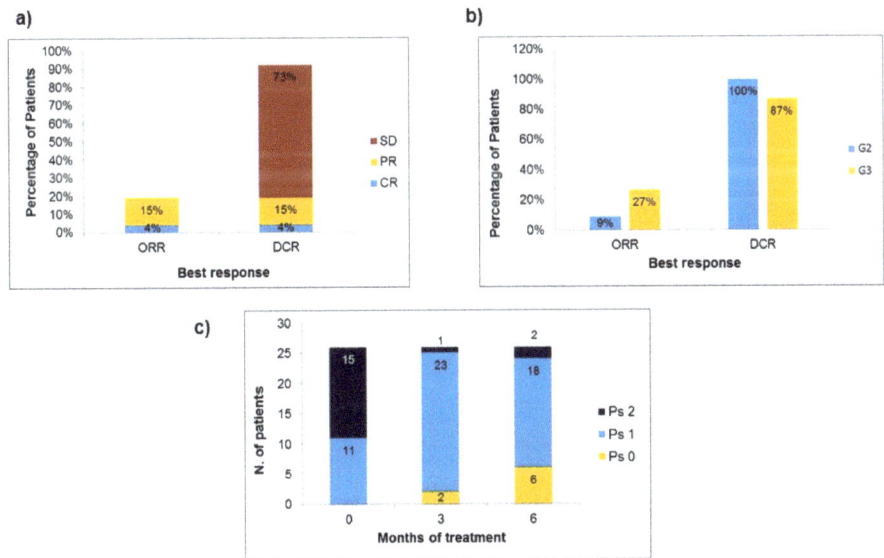

Figure 1. Histogram representations of activity and clinical benefit of mTMZ. Response rates with mTMZ in all patients (**a**) and according to grading (G2 vs. G3) of the tumor (**b**). Improvement of ECOG PS over 3 and 6 months of treatment (**c**). CR = Complete Response; DCR = Disease Control Rate; ORR = Overall Response Rate; PR = Partial Response; PS = Performance Status; SD = Stable Disease.

The overall DCR was 92%. The ORR and DCR in patients with G2 NENs were 9% and 100%, respectively, while for those with G3 NENs the ORR was 27% and the DCR was 87% (Figure 1b). A clinical improvement of the basal PS was reported in 73% of patients (Figure 1c). The mPFS was 9 months and longer for patients with G2 NENs (mPFS: 23.6 months) compared to patients with G3 NENs (mPFS: 8.9 months), although not significant ($p = 0.16$) (Figure 2).

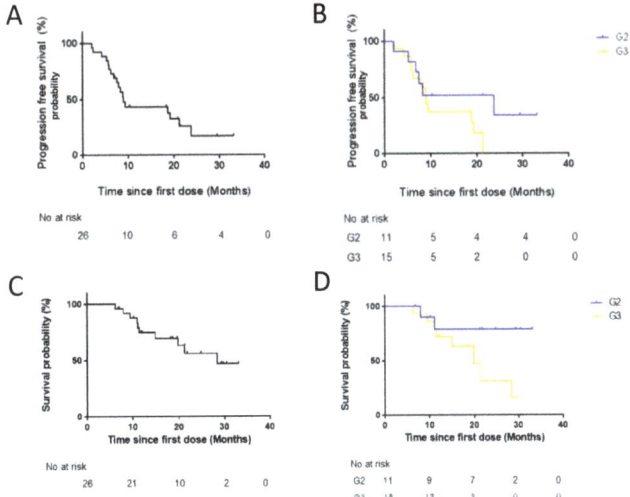

Figure 2. Time-to-outcome analyses. Curves of progression-free survival and overall survival in all patients (**A,C**) and according to grading (**B,D**).

The mOS was 28.3 months in the entire population. The mOS was 19.8 months in patients with G3 NENs and not reached in patient with G2 NENs ($p = 0.60$) (Figure 2). No G3/G4 toxicities were registered (Table 3); no dose reductions were reported. The two most common adverse events were anemia and asthenia (Table 3). The median time-on-TMZ therapy was 12.2 months (95% CI: 11.4–19.6). No patient discontinued treatment for the occurrence of severe adverse events.

Table 3. Summary of adverse events.

Toxicity	G1		G2		G3/G4	
	No	%	No	%	No	%
Anaemia	11	42.3	13	50.0	0	0.0
Asthenia	9	34.6	12	46.1	0	0.0
Neuropathy	8	30.7	10	38.4	0	0.0
Neutropenia	8	30.7	8	30.7	0	0.0
Nausea	7	26.9	8	30.7	0	0.0
Hyperbilirubinemia	7	26.9	6	23.1	0	0.0
Alkaline phosphatase	3	11.5	0	0.0	0	0.0
Hyperglycaemia	4	15.3	6	23.1	0	0.0
Thrombocytopenia	0	0.0	6	23.1	0	0.0

4. Discussion

Currently, the optimal schedule for TMZ has still not been established. Different schedules have been used in recent trials both in monotherapy and in association with other drugs [6–16]; these studies were heterogeneous in terms of sample size, histology, grading, and number and type of previous treatments (Table S1 in Supplementary Material). Although a significant activity was constantly reported with these schedules, the median time on TMZ was negatively influenced by G3/G4 toxicities [6,13,16] with a discontinuation rate up to 55%. This highlights the need to minimize toxicity. To this regard, albeit retrospective and exploratory, we report the first "hypothesis generating" study with mTMZ 75mg/m^2 "one week on-one week off" scheme in NENs. The treatment was associated with an ORR of 19% and an overall DCR of 92%; most importantly, no G3/G4 adverse events and no interruptions of treatment for toxicity were registered. In addition, mTMZ determined a clinical benefit through improvement of PS.

Notably, there were no significant relationships between response to therapy and characteristics of patients and disease, including age (≤65 vs. >65 years), sex (male vs. female), PS ECOG (1 vs. 2), site of primary tumor [gastro-intestinal (GI) vs. no-GI], KI-67 level (<20 vs. ≥20%), grading (G2 vs. G3), number of metastatic sites (1 vs. 2 vs. ≥3) and previous treatments (see Table S2 in Supplementary Material). However, we cannot rule out the hypothesis that such evaluations could be affected by the small sample size of our series. In fact, although not significant, responses were more frequently observed in G3 NENs (4 pts) compared to G2 (1 patient). It is well known that grade is associated with cell proliferation rate which is a consistent indicator of chemosensitivity. Unfortunately, high grade tumors are in turn characterized by high genomic heterogeneity with frequent p53, Hedgehog and Notch mutations [26] (associated to drug resistance and plasticity of stem-*like* states), and after an initial response to therapy, they acquire a drug resistant phenotype in a short time. For this reason, very frequently, a discrepancy is observed between higher response rates and shorter progression-free survival in G3 NENs, as occurs in our series.

The clinical advantages of a low-dose administration of TMZ have been explored over the last 20 years and are mainly based on (i) a lower toxicity profile eventually associated (ii) to a better quality of life [27–30]. An important characteristic of our series was the inclusion of 15 pts with PS ECOG 2 (57.7%) while in previous trials it ranged from 0 to 28% (Table S1 in Supplementary Material). Interestingly, mTMZ was well-tolerated, without any G3/G4 adverse effects, and in 14 out of 15 pts there was an improvement of PS 2 to PS 1 after 3 months of therapy. This suggests that mTMZ might be given to patients with deteriorated PS when the benefit-risk balance is not favorable for more aggressive treatments.

Furthermore, beyond these clinical advantages, mTMZ, but not the conventional scheme, is able to trigger anti-angiogenetic and immune-mediated pathways [17–23]. NENs are hypervascularised tumors and overexpress a plethora of proangiogenic molecules and related receptors [31–35]. Therefore, given their high dependence from angiogenic pathways, the metronomic schedule, through its predominant anti-angiogenic action, could represent a stronger candidate for NENs treatment. Additionally, metronomic therapy exerts its anti-angiogenetic activity through the increase of the inhibitor thrombospodin-1 (THBS-1) and the inhibition of the hypoxia-inducible factor 1 (HIF-1) [36]. These biologic properties account for a *more* potent and clinically relevant anti-angiogenic than cytotoxic effect of mTMZ. Furthermore, these latter effects could be particularly interesting for combination with mTOR inhibitors (i.e., everolimus). Inhibition of mTORC1 (mTOR Complex 1) causes the loss of a negative feedback loop that activates HIF-1 [37]; therefore, the association of an mTOR inhibitor with mTMZ might preserve the anti-angiogenic activity of this loop.

Notably, the evaluation of O6-methylguanine DNA methyltransferase (MGMT), which repairs the methylation at the O6-position of guanine induced by alkylating agents [38–41] did not show to be significant in our series. Our group is going to accumulate more data about this issue. On the basis of these clinical results and to further investigate the role of mTMZ in second-line treatment of G3 NENs, a study is currently ongoing at the ENETS center of Naples. This larger and prospective clinical trial named TENEC trial (TEmozolomide in NeuroEndocrine Carcinoma), is supported by ITANET (ITalian Association for NEuroendocrine Tumors) and aims to confirm the efficacy and toxicity results of mTMZ as well as its modulating effects on host' immune system.

Despite the exploratory and retrospective nature of our study, the efficacy of mTMZ in monotherapy here reported is similar to that shown in other retrospective trials with conventional schedules of TMZ monotherapy; conversely, the toxicity profile is clearly better.

5. Conclusions

Our study is a proof of concept that an intermittent schedule of mTMZ at 75 mg/m^2 can be an effective treatment in advanced G2-3 NENs, a suitable therapeutic option for PS 2 patients as well as a strong candidate also for combination treatments.

Supplementary Materials: The following are available online at http://www.mdpi.com/2077-0383/8/8/1224/s1, Table S1: Characteristics of studies reporting outcomes of TMZ in NENs, Table S2: Clinico–pathological characteristics of patients according to treatment response.

Author Contributions: Conceptualization, A.O., C.v.A., S.T., A.C.; methodology, A.O. and M.C.; validation, C.v.A., M.C., M.M., F.T., S.T.; formal analysis, A.O., M.C. and C.v.A.; investigation, A.C., S.T., C.v.A., M.C., R.M., M.M., F.T., M.L.B., M.L.T., A.D.S.; data curation, C.v.A. and A.C.; writing and original draft preparation, A.O., M.C., S.T., C.v.A.

Funding: This research was funded by Lega Italiana per la Lotta contro i Tumori (LILT), Naples section.

Acknowledgments: We thank Alessandra Trocino, Librarian at the Library of Istituto Nazionale Tumori Fondazione 'G Pascale', Naples, Italy, for her excellent bibliographic service and assistance.

Conflicts of Interest: The authors declare no conflict of interest.

References

1. Dasari, A.; Shen, C.; Halperin, D.; Zhao, B.; Zhou, S.; Xu, Y.; Shih, T.; Yao, J.C. Trends in the Incidence, Prevalence, and Survival Outcomes in Patients with Neuroendocrine Tumors in the United States. *JAMA Oncol.* **2017**, *3*, 1335–1342. [CrossRef] [PubMed]
2. National Comprehensive Cancer Network. Neuroendocrine and Adrenal Tumor (Version 2.2018). Available online: https://www.nccn.org/professionals/physician_gls/PDF/neuroendocrine.pdf (accessed on 2 August 2019).

3. Hallet, J.; Law, C.H.; Cukier, M.; Saskin, R.; Liu, N.; Singh, S. Exploring the rising incidence of neuroendocrine tumors: A population–based analysis of epidemiology, metastatic presentation, and outcomes. *Cancer* **2015**, *121*, 589–597. [CrossRef] [PubMed]
4. Pavel, M.; Costa, F.; Capdevila, J.; Gross, D.; Kianmanesh, R.; Krenning, E.; Knigge, U.; Salazar, R.; Pape, U.F.; Öberg, K. ENETS Consensus Guidelines Update for the Management of Distant Metastatic Disease of Intestinal, Pancreatic, Bronchial Neuroendocrine Neoplasms (NEN) and NEN of Unknown Primary Site. *Neuroendocrinology* **2016**, *103*, 172–185. [CrossRef] [PubMed]
5. Strosberg, J.R.; Halfdanarson, T.R.; Bellizzi, A.M.; Chan, J.A.; Dillon, J.S.; Heaney, A.P.; Kunz, P.L.; O'Dorisio, T.M.; Salem, R.; Segelov, E.; et al. The North American Neuroendocrine Tumor Society Consensus Guidelines for Surveillance and Medical Management of Midgut Neuroendocrine Tumors. *Pancreas* **2017**, *46*, 707–714. [CrossRef] [PubMed]
6. Ekeblad, S.; Sundin, A.; Janson, E.T.; Welin, S.; Granberg, D.; Kindmark, H.; Dunder, K.; Kozlovacki, G.; Örlefors, H.; Sigurd, M.; et al. Temozolomide as monotherapy is effective in treatment of advanced malignant neuroendocrine tumors. *Clin. Cancer Res.* **2007**, *13*, 2986–2991. [CrossRef] [PubMed]
7. Olsen, I.H.; Sørensen, J.B.; Federspiel, B.; Kjaer, A.; Hansen, C.P.; Knigge, U.; Langer, S.W. Temozolomide as second or third line treatment of patients with neuroendocrine carcinomas. *Sci. World J.* **2012**, *2012*, 170496. [CrossRef] [PubMed]
8. Strosberg, J.R.; Fine, R.L.; Choi, J.; Nasir, A.; Coppola, D.; Chen, D.T.; Helm, J.; Kvols, L. First-line chemotherapy with capecitabine and temozolomide in patients with metastatic pancreatic endocrine carcinomas. *Cancer* **2011**, *117*, 268–275. [CrossRef]
9. Welin, S.; Sorbye, H.; Sebjornsen, S.; Knappskog, S.; Busch, C.; Öberg, K. Clinical effect of temozolomide–based chemotherapy in poorly differentiated endocrine carcinoma after progression on first–line chemotherapy. *Cancer* **2011**, *117*, 4617–4622. [CrossRef]
10. Saif, M.W.; Kaley, K.; Brennan, M.; Garcon, M.C.; Rodriguez, G.; Rodriguez, T. A retrospective study of capecitabine/temozolomide (CAPTEM) regimen in the treatment of metastatic pancreatic neuroendocrine tumors (pNETs) after failing previous therapy. *JOP* **2013**, *14*, 498–501.
11. Fine, R.L.; Gulati, A.P.; Krantz, B.A.; Moss, R.A.; Schreibman, S.; Tsushima, D.A.; Mowatt, K.B.; Dinnen, R.D.; Mao, Y.; Stevens, P.D.; et al. Capecitabine and temozolomide (CAPTEM) for metastatic, well–differentiated neuroendocrine cancers: The Pancreas Center at Columbia University experience. *Cancer Chemother. Pharmacol.* **2013**, *71*, 663–670. [CrossRef]
12. Saranga–Perry, V.; Morse, B.; Centeno, B.; Kvols, L.; Strosberg, J. Treatment of metastatic neuroendocrine tumors of the thymus with capecitabine and temozolomide: A case series. *Neuroendocrinology* **2013**, *97*, 318–321. [CrossRef] [PubMed]
13. Chan, J.A.; Blaszkowsky, L.; Stuart, K.; Zhu, A.X.; Allen, J.; Wadlow, R.; Ryan, D.P.; Meyerhardt, J.; Gonzalez, M.; Regan, E.; et al. A prospective, phase 1/2 study of everolimus and temozolomide in patients with advanced pancreatic neuroendocrine tumor. *Cancer* **2013**, *119*, 3212–3218. [CrossRef] [PubMed]
14. Koumarianou, A.; Antoniou, S.; Kanakis, G.; Economopoulos, N.; Rontogianni, D.; Ntavatzikos, A.; Tsavaris, N.; Pectasides, D.; Dimitriadis, G.; Kaltsas, G. Combination treatment with metronomic temozolomide, bevacizumab and long–acting octreotide for malignant neuroendocrine tumors. *Endocr. Relat. Cancer* **2012**, *19*, L1–L4. [CrossRef] [PubMed]
15. Chan, J.A.; Stuart, K.; Earle, C.C.; Clark, J.W.; Bhargava, P.; Miksad, R.; Blaszkowsky, L.; Enzinger, P.C.; Meyerhardt, J.A.; Zheng, H.; et al. Prospective study of bevacizumab plus temozolomide in patients with advanced neuroendocrine tumors. *J. Clin. Oncol.* **2012**, *30*, 2963–2968. [CrossRef] [PubMed]
16. Kulke, M.H.; Stuart, K.; Enzinger, P.C.; Ryan, D.P.; Clark, J.W.; Muzikansky, A.; Vincitore, M.; Michelini, A.; Fuchs, C.S. Phase II study of temozolomide and thalidomide in patients with metastatic neuroendocrine tumors. *J. Clin. Oncol.* **2006**, *24*, 401–406. [CrossRef] [PubMed]
17. Kurzen, H.; Schmitt, S.; Näher, H.; Möhler, T. Inhibition of angiogenesis by non–toxic doses of temozolomide. *Anticancer Drugs* **2003**, *14*, 515–522. [CrossRef] [PubMed]
18. Sun, C.; Yu, Y.; Wang, L.; Wu, B.; Xia, L.; Feng, F.; Ling, Z.; Wang, S. Additive antiangiogenesis effect of ginsenoside Rg3 with low–dose metronomic temozolomide on rat glioma cells both in vivo and in vitro. *J. Exp. Clin. Cancer Res.* **2016**, *35*, 32. [CrossRef] [PubMed]

19. Woo, J.Y.; Yang, S.H.; Lee, Y.S.; Lee, S.Y.; Kim, J.; Hong, Y.K. Continuous Low–Dose Temozolomide Chemotherapy and Microvessel Density in Recurrent Glioblastoma. *J. Korean Neurosurg. Soc.* **2015**, *58*, 426–431. [CrossRef]
20. Kaneno, R.; Shurin, G.V.; Tourkova, I.L.; Shurin, M.R. Chemomodulation of human dendritic cell function by antineoplastic agents in low noncytotoxic concentrations. *J. Transl. Med.* **2009**, *7*, 58. [CrossRef]
21. Ghiringhelli, F.; Menard, C.; Puig, P.E.; Ladoire, S.; Roux, S.; Martin, F.; Solary, E.; Le Cesne, A.; Zitvogel, L.; Chauffert, B. Metronomic cyclophosphamide regimen selectively depletes CD4$^+$CD25$^+$ regulatory T cells and restores T and NK effector functions in end stage cancer patients. *Cancer Immunol. Immunother.* **2007**, *56*, 641–648. [CrossRef]
22. Banissi, C.; Ghiringhelli, F.; Chen, L.; Carpentier, A.F. Treg depletion with a lowdose metronomic temozolomide regimen in a rat glioma model. *Cancer Immunol. Immunother.* **2009**, *58*, 1627–1634. [CrossRef] [PubMed]
23. Zhao, J.; Cao, Y.; Lei, Z.; Yang, Z.; Zhang, B.; Huang, B. Selective depletion of CD4$^+$CD25$^+$Foxp3$^+$ regulatory T cells by low–dose cyclophosphamide is explained by reduced intracellular ATP levels. *Cancer Res.* **2010**, *70*, 4850–4858. [CrossRef] [PubMed]
24. Kan, S.; Hazama, S.; Maeda, K.; Inoue, Y.; Homma, S.; Koido, S.; Okamoto, M.; Oka, M. Suppressive Effects of Cyclophosphamide and Gemcitabine on Regulatory T–Cell Induction In Vitro. *Anticancer Res.* **2012**, *32*, 5363–5369. [PubMed]
25. National Institute of Health. Available online: https://ctep.cancer.gov/protocolDevelopment/electronic_applications/ctc.htm#ctc_40 (accessed on 2 August 2019).
26. Girardi, D.M.; Silva, A.C.B.; Rêgo, J.F.M.; Coudry, R.A.; Riechelmann, R.P. Unraveling molecular pathways of poorly differentiated neuroendocrine carcinomas of the gastroenteropancreatic system: A systematic review. *Cancer Treat. Rev.* **2017**, *56*, 28–35. [CrossRef] [PubMed]
27. Fidler, I.J.; Ellis, L.M. Chemotherapeutic drugs—More really is not better. *Nat. Med.* **2000**, *6*, 500–502. [CrossRef]
28. Gatenby, R.A.; Silva, A.S.; Gillies, R.J.; Frieden, B.R. Adaptive Therapy. *Cancer Res.* **2009**, *69*, 4894–4903. [CrossRef]
29. Scharovsky, O.G.; Mainetti, L.E.; Rozados, V.R. Metronomic chemotherapy: Changing the paradigm that more is better. *Curr. Oncol.* **2009**, *16*, 7–15. [CrossRef]
30. Pasquier, E.; Kavallaris, M.; André, N. Metronomic chemotherapy: New rationale for new directions. *Nat. Rev. Clin. Oncol.* **2010**, *7*, 455–465. [CrossRef]
31. Scoazec, J.Y. Angiogenesis in neuroendocrine tumors: Therapeutic applications. *Neuroendocrinology* **2013**, *97*, 45–56. [CrossRef]
32. Besig, S.; Voland, P.; Baur, D.M.; Perren, A.; Prinz, C. Vascular endothelial growth factors, angiogenesis, and survival in human ileal enterochromaffin cell carcinoids. *Neuroendocrinology* **2009**, *90*, 402–415. [CrossRef]
33. Zhang, J.; Jia, Z.; Li, Q.; Wang, L.; Rashid, A.; Zhu, Z.; Evans, D.B.; Vauthey, J.N.; Xie, K.; Yao, J.C. Elevated expression of vascular endothelial growth factor correlates with increased angiogenesis and decreased progression–free survival among patients with low–grade neuroendocrine tumors. *Cancer* **2007**, *109*, 1478–1486. [CrossRef] [PubMed]
34. Zhou, Q.; Guo, P.; Wang, X.; Nuthalapati, S.; Gallo, J.M. Preclinical pharmacokinetic and pharmacodynamic evaluation of metronomic and conventional temozolomide dosing regimens. *J. Pharmacol. Exp. Ther.* **2007**, *321*, 265–275. [CrossRef] [PubMed]
35. Lambrescu, I.; Fica, S.; Martins, D.; Spada, F.; Cella, C.; Bertani, E.; Rubino, M.; Gibelli, B.; Grana, C.; Bonomo, G.; et al. Metronomic and metronomic–like therapies in neuroendocrine tumors—Rationale and clinical perspectives. *Cancer Treat. Rev.* **2017**, *55*, 46–56. [CrossRef] [PubMed]
36. André, N.; Carré, M.; Pasquier, E. Metronomics: Towards personalized chemotherapy? *Nat. Rev. Clin. Oncol.* **2014**, *11*, 413–431. [CrossRef] [PubMed]
37. Figlin, R.A.; Kaufmann, I.; Brechbiel, J. Targeting PI3K and mTORC2 in metastatic renal cell carcinoma: New strategies for overcoming resistance to VEGFR and mTORC1 inhibitors. *Int. J. Cancer* **2013**, *133*, 788–796. [CrossRef] [PubMed]
38. Schmitt, A.M.; Pavel, M.; Rudolph, T.; Dawson, H.; Blank, A.; Komminoth, P.; Vassella, E.; Perren, A. Prognostic and predictive roles of MGMT protein expression and promoter methylation in sporadic pancreatic neuroendocrine neoplasms. *Neuroendocrinology* **2014**, *100*, 35–44. [CrossRef] [PubMed]

39. Walter, T.; van Brakel, B.; Vercherat, C.; Hervieu, V.; Forestier, J.; Chayvialle, J.A. O6–Methylguanine–DNA methyltransferase status in neuroendocrine tumors: Prognostic relevance and association with response to alkylating agents. *Br. J. Cancer* **2015**, *112*, 523–531. [CrossRef]
40. Kulke, M.H.; Hornick, J.L.; Frauenhoffer, C.; Hooshmand, S.; Ryan, D.P.; Enzinger, P.C.; Meyerhardt, J.A.; Clark, J.W.; Stuart, K.; Fuchs, C.S.; et al. O6–methylguanine DNA methyltransferase deficiency and response to temozolomide–based therapy in patients with neuroendocrine tumors. *Clin. Cancer Res.* **2009**, *15*, 338–345. [CrossRef]
41. Raj, N.; Klimstra, D.S.; Horvat, N.; Zhang, L.; Chou, J.F.; Capanu, M.; Basturk, O.; Do, R.K.G.; Allen, P.J.; Reidy-Lagunes, D. O6–Methylguanine DNA Methyltransferase Status Does Not Predict Response or Resistance to Alkylating Agents in Well–Differentiated Pancreatic Neuroendocrine Tumors. *Pancreas* **2017**, *46*, 758–763. [CrossRef]

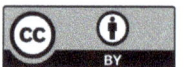

© 2019 by the authors. Licensee MDPI, Basel, Switzerland. This article is an open access article distributed under the terms and conditions of the Creative Commons Attribution (CC BY) license (http://creativecommons.org/licenses/by/4.0/).

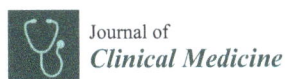

Article

Multidisciplinary Management of Neuroendocrine Neoplasia: A Real-World Experience from a Referral Center

Ludovica Magi [1], Federica Mazzuca [2,3], Maria Rinzivillo [1], Giulia Arrivi [2], Emanuela Pilozzi [3,4], Daniela Prosperi [5], Elsa Iannicelli [6,7], Paolo Mercantini [7,8], Michele Rossi [6,7], Patrizia Pizzichini [5], Andrea Laghi [6,7], Alberto Signore [5,7], Paolo Marchetti [2,3], Bruno Annibale [1,7] and Francesco Panzuto [1,*]

1. Digestive Disease Unit, ENETS Center of Excellence, Sant'Andrea University Hospital, 00189 Rome, Italy; ludovicamagi@hotmail.it (L.M.); mariarinzivillo@gmail.com (M.R.); Bruno.annibale@uniroma1.it (B.A.)
2. Medical Oncology Unit, ENETS Center of Excellence, Sant'Andrea University Hospital, 00189 Rome, Italy; federica.mazzuca@uniroma1.it (F.M.); giulia.arrivi@uniroma1.it (G.A.); Paolo.marchetti@uniroma1.it (P.M.)
3. Department of Clinical and Molecular Medicine, "Sapienza" University of Rome, 00189 Rome, Italy; Emanuela.pilozzi@uniroma1.it
4. Pathologic Anatomy and Molecular Morphology Unit, ENETS Center of Excellence, Sant'Andrea University Hospital, 00189 Rome, Italy
5. Nuclear Medicine Unit, ENETS Center of Excellence, Sant'Andrea University Hospital, 00189 Rome, Italy; Dprosperi@ospedalesantandrea.it (D.P.); ppizzichini@ospedalesantandrea.it (P.P.); alberto.signore@uniroma1.it (A.S.)
6. Radiology Unit, ENETS Center of Excellence, Sant'Andrea University Hospital, 00189 Rome, Italy; Elsa.iannicelli@uniroma1.it (E.I.); Michele.rossi@uniroma1.it (M.R.); Andrea.laghi@uniroma1.it (A.L.)
7. Department of Medical-Surgical Sciences and Translational Medicine, "Sapienza" University of Rome, 00189 Rome, Italy; Paolo.mercantini@uniroma1.it
8. Surgery Unit, ENETS Center of Excellence, Sant'Andrea University Hospital, 00189 Rome, Italy
* Correspondence: fpanzuto@ospedalesantandrea.it

Received: 27 May 2019; Accepted: 21 June 2019; Published: 25 June 2019

Abstract: Purpose: Multidisciplinary approach is widely advised for an effective care of patients with neuroendocrine neoplasia (NEN). Since data on efficacy of multidisciplinary management of NENs patients in referral centers are scanty, this study aimed at analyzing the modality of presentation and clinical outcome of patients with NENs managed by a dedicated multidisciplinary team. Methods. In this prospective observational study, we included all consecutive new patients visiting the Sant'Andrea Hospital in Rome (ENETS—Center of Excellence) between January 2014 and June 2018. Results. A total of 195 patients were evaluated. The most frequent sites were pancreas (38.5%), small bowel (22%), and lung (9.7%). Median Ki67 was 3%. After the first visit at the center, additional radiological and/or nuclear medicine procedures were requested in 163 patients (83.6%), whereas histological data revision was advised in 84 patients (43.1%) (revision of histological slides: 27.7%, new bioptic sampling: 15.4%). After that, disease imaging staging and grading was modified in 30.7% and 17.9% of patients, respectively. Overall, a change in therapeutic management was proposed in 98 patients (50.3%). Conclusions. Multidisciplinary approach in a dedicated team may lead to change of disease imaging staging and grading in a significant proportion of patients. Enhancing referral routes to dedicated-NEN center should be promoted, since it may improve patients' clinical outcome.

Keywords: neuroendocrine tumors; multidisciplinary; management; outcome; grading; staging

1. Introduction

Neuroendocrine neoplasia (NEN) is a group of rare and heterogenous diseases, in terms of both pathological and clinical features. Their prognosis is affected by several factors, including primary tumor site, staging, and grading [1–3]. They promise a clinical challenge for physicians, because they may have various growth patterns ranging from very slowly progressive to rapidly aggressive tumors. An effective diagnosis of NEN is based on clinical presentation, pathology, cross-sectional imaging (computed tomography (CT) or magnetic resonance imaging (MRI)), and functional nuclear medicine procedures, including 68-Gallium PET and 18FDG PET [4–6]. Recently, the involvement of the immune system and the role of tumor micro-environment has also been suggested as important in tumor evolution [7]. Surgery is widely considered the sole chance to cure patients; however, it is often not feasible due to advanced metastatic disease at time of diagnosis. In these patients, for whom medical treatment is required, several therapeutic options are available, including somatostatin analogs (octreotide and lanreotide), peptide receptor radionuclide therapy (PRRT), targeted therapies (everolimus and sunitinib), and systemic chemotherapy [4].

Due to the complexity of NEN management, a multidisciplinary approach is widely advised for an effective care of patients with this uncommon kind of cancer. Multidisciplinary care is strongly encouraged by both the European and North American Neuroendocrine Tumor Society [8,9]. There has been some evidence of better survival in patients managed in centers with dedicated multidisciplinary team (MDT) compared to those treated with standard care in different kinds of cancers [10,11]. However, the real impact of MDT on patients' survival may vary depending on structural and functional components and the expertise of the participants [12]. Since data on the efficacy of multidisciplinary management of patients with NENs in specialized centers with dedicated MDT are scanty, this study aimed at analyzing the modalities of presentation and clinical outcome of patients with NENs managed in a center of excellence with a dedicated MDT.

2. Patients and Methods

This is a prospective observational study including all consecutive new patients visiting the Sant'Andrea Hospital site of Rome (part of the Rome ENETS Center of Excellence) between January 2014 and June 2018. In accordance with the center standard of procedures, all major clinical and pathological data were collected in a computer anonymized database. All patients were discussed in an NEN multidisciplinary team that included several clinicians involved in patients' management: oncologist, gastroenterologist, surgeon, nuclear medicine physician, radiologist, and pathologist.

Based on data retrieved from available charts, gastrointestinal and pancreatic NENs were retrospectively classified according to WHO 2010 [13] and WHO 2017 [14] classifications, whereas the WHO 2014 [15] classification was used for lung NENs. Tumor grading was assessed according to the ENETS grading system in gastro-entero-pancreatic (GEP) NENs, as well as in lung NENs [1,16,17]. Pathological revision was performed in those patients for whom available histological information was not accurate enough to obtain an NEN diagnosis in accordance with ENETS standards of care [18]. When required, repeating bioptic sampling was proposed to the patients after MDT discussion. Patients' follow-up was performed in accordance with ENETS recommendations [19].

The distribution of continuous variables was reported as the median and interquartile range (IQR; 25th–75th percentiles) or range, as appropriate. A comparison between the subgroups was carried out using Fisher's exact test or the chi-square test for noncontinuous variables, whereas the Mann–Whitney U test was used to compare the non-normally distributed continuous independent variables, as appropriate. Overall survival analysis was performed using the Kaplan–Meier method. This work was carried out in accordance with the Declaration of Helsinki. Full informed consent for data collection was obtained from all patients.

3. Results

A total of 318 patients were evaluated. Of these, 123 patients (38.7%) were excluded because they had been referred to the center with the intention of obtaining a second opinion (Figure 1); since these patients were not taken in care by the center, no data on their follow-up were available. Thus, final analysis was performed on 195 patients, including 94 males (48.2%), with a median age of 59 years (IQR 51–70.5 years). Of these, 163 patients had GEP NENs (83.6%) and 19 patients had lung primary NEN (9.7%). In the remaining 13 patients (6.7%), the primary tumor site was unknown (Table 1).

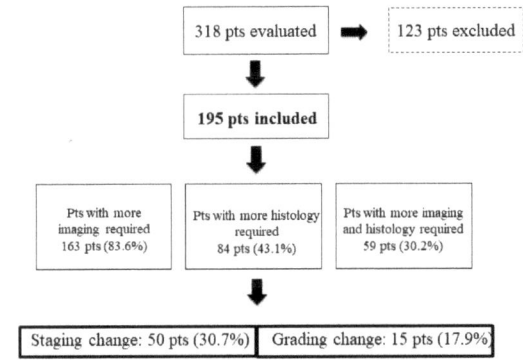

Figure 1. Staging and grading modification after visit at the Center. pts, patients.

Table 1. Patients' general features.

	Overall n = 195	Newly Diagnosed n = 48	Referred n = 147	p-Value
Primary site				
Pancreas	75 (38.5%)	22 (45.8%)	53 (36%)	
Small bowel	43 (22.1%)	10 (20.8%)	33 (22.4%)	
Rectum	10 (5.1%)	2 (4.2%)	8 (5.4%)	0.642
Appendix	9 (4.6%)	2 (4.2%)	7 (4.7%)	
Lung	19 (9.7%)	6 (12.5%)	13 (8.8%)	
Other	39 (20%)	6 (12.5%)	33 (22.4%)	
Grading				
G1	88 (45.1%)	22 (45.8%)	66 (44.9%)	
G2	80 (41%)	18 (37.5%)	62 (42.2%)	0.053
G3	27 (13.9%)	8 (16.7%)	19 (12.9%)	
Median Ki67 (IQR, range)	3% (2–9, 1–90)	2% (2–5, 1–40)	3% (2–10, 1–90)	0.212
Staging				
Stage 1	42 (21.5%)	13 (27.1%)	29 (19.7%)	
Stage 2	27 (13.9%)	6 (12.5%)	21 (14.3%)	0.080
Stage 3	38 (19.5%)	8 (16.7%)	30 (20.4%)	
Stage 4	88 (45.1%)	21 (43.7%)	67 (45.6%)	

At time of initial visit at the center, the Ki67 value was available in 177 patients (90.8%), the median value being 3% (IQR 2–9). All but 7 patients (96.4%) had tumors with well differentiated morphology.

Overall, 147 patients (75.4%) already had NEN diagnosis at time of referral; in these patients, the median interval between initial NEN diagnosis and time of referral to the center was 4 months (IQR 2–13.5 months). The remaining 48 patients (24.6%) were newly diagnosed at the center. Patients' general features are summarized in Table 1. Overall, 68 patients (34.8%) were discussed multiple times by MDT after initial evaluation.

A total of 63 patients (32.3%) got in touch with the center using the center's website form, whereas 132 patients (67.7%) booked the first visit through public health regional system tools (dedicated phone number, direct hospital access). Seventy-four patients (37.9%) were referred to the center by other hospitals. The median waiting time to obtain the first visit in the NEN-dedicated ambulatory was 7 days (IQR 7–10 days).

Patients' Management

After first visit, additional cross-sectional radiological examinations and/or nuclear medicine diagnostic procedures were requested in 163 patients (83.6%) (Figure 1). In particular, CT or MRI was prescribed in 123 patients (63.1%) (additional CT or MR was considered to be necessary, because either a new updated staging was necessary or CT/MR had not been previously performed or they were of insufficient image quality or incomplete according to the imaging standard of our center), ^{68}Ga-DOTA-NOC Positron Emission Tomography (PET)/CT in 107 patients (54.9%) (resulting positive in 83 of them, 77.7%), and (^{18}F)FDG PET/CT in 42 patients (21.5%) (resulting positive in 15 of them, 35.7%). Dual PET/CT, with ^{68}Ga-DOTA-NOC and (^{18}F) fluorodeoxyglucose (FDG), were performed in 21 patients (10.8%). Overall, a positive finding was observed in 65% of patients for whom an additional functional imaging procedure (^{68}Ga-DOTA-NOC or (^{18}F)FDG-PET) was requested.

After evaluating the requested radiological/nuclear medicine procedures, a change in disease staging was performed in 50/163 patients (30.7%).

Integration of available pathological data was advised in 84 patients (43.1%) (Figure 1). Specifically, revision of available histological slides was required in 54 patients (27.7%), whereas new bioptic sampling was performed in 30 patients (15.4%). Pathological revision consisted of histology in all but 2 patients, in whom cytology was performed. After histological data integration, pathological change in terms of grading modification was observed in 15 patients (17.9%). Specifically, a grading increase was observed in 10 patients (5 patients moved from G1 to G2, 5 patients from G2 to G3), whereas a grading decrease was observed in the remaining 5 patients (from G2 to G1).

A total of 174 patients (89.2%) received a decision concerning subsequent follow-up within 1 month after their initial visit at the center. All suggestions proposed by the MDTs were executed. Overall, a change in clinical management was proposed in 98 patients (50.3%). Of these, 67 patients (68.4%) received medical treatment (changes in medical treatments after first MDT discussion are detailed in Table 2) (most frequently somatostatin analogs (37 patients, 37.8%); followed by everolimus (15 patients, 15.3%), systemic chemotherapy (6 patients, 6.1%), sunitinib (5 patients, 2.7%), and peptide receptor radionuclide therapy (4 patients 4%). Nine patients (9.2%) underwent surgery, and 19 patients (19.4%) were followed up without medical or surgical intervention.

Table 2. Changes in medical treatments after first multidisciplinary discussion.

	Before MDT *	After MDT
Somatostatin analogs	23 (11.8%)	37 (19%)
Targeted therapies	3 (1.5%)	20 (10.3%)
Peptide receptor radionuclide therapy	1 (0.5%)	4 (2%)
Systemic chemotherapy	26 (13.3%)	6 (3%)

* 14/67 patients were not receiving medical treatment before discussion.

A total of 28 patients (14.4%) died of disease during a median follow-up period of 17 months (IQR 7.2–33 months) after initial diagnosis at the center. Median survival after initial diagnosis at the center was not reached, whereas 5-y survival rate was 62.6%. Median survival in stage IV patients was 59 months.

4. Discussion

Although several studies have demonstrated a potential positive impact on patients' clinical care in different kinds of cancers, it has been recently suggested that tumor boards are only as good as their structural and functional components and the expertise of the participants [12]. As far as NENs are concerned, knowledge of MDT impact on patients' care is even scantier [20–22]. International guidelines for NENs emphasize collaboration among diverse medical disciplines to improve patients' care and standardize diagnostic and therapeutic approaches. However, despite the widespread use of multidisciplinary teams for the management of NEN patients in the clinical practice, few data on their effect on care exist.

The present study reports the real-world experience of a referral center in which, according with the ENETS standard of procedures, newly patients are routinely discussed in a multidisciplinary setting. Interestingly, almost 2/3 of patients included presented with advanced disease at time of initial referral, stage 3 and 4 being observed in 19.5% and 45.1%, respectively, or with tumor with moderate-high proliferative activity, with the G2 and G3 group representing 41% and 13.9%, respectively. In accordance with other series [23,24], this figure confirms that NEN patients presenting to a referral center often have advanced, progressive disease requiring specific diagnostic investigations and tailored therapeutic approaches that need to be shared in a multidisciplinary discussion.

In the present study, most patients (75.4%) referred to the center with NEN had already been diagnosed at the time of center referral, with the median interval between initial diagnosis and center referral being 4 months (IQR 2–13.5). Almost all patients (89.2%) received decision concerning subsequent follow-up within 1 month after their initial visit. Prompt multidisciplinary evaluation helps to expedite the beginning of optimal therapeutic strategy in NEN patients, which may result in a more favorable clinical outcome. Recent studies reported a long interval varying from 24 to 53.8 months from onset of symptoms and definitive diagnosis in NEN patients, leading to a delayed diagnosis and a plausible worse overall prognosis [25]. Early referral to an NEN-dedicated center may give patients a higher probability to receive prompt accurate disease staging, a tailored therapeutic approach, and may result in a better chance to participate in clinical trials, an option which is considered the best management opportunity to be especially encouraged (NCCN Guidelines, www.nccn.org).

After referral to the center, integration or revision of pathological data was advised in a significant proportion of patients (43.1%), because available data were considered not accurate enough in accordance with the ENETS standards of care [18], with new bioptic sampling being advised in 15.4% of patients. In accordance with data obtained by pathological data integration/revision, a grading change occurred in 17.9% of patients. It is well known that grading is the most powerful prognostic factor in NENs and may be considered a decision-driving marker when planning treatment [2,3,26–28]. Tumor grading needs to be assessed by evaluating the Ki67 proliferation index, and the number of counted cells (recommended 500 to 2000) has to be mentioned [29]. Clinicians dealing with NEN patients should always check whether the pathology report includes an accurate grading assessment, otherwise pathological data revision or integration by repeating tumor biopsy is advocated. Since there is the possibility of Ki67 changes throughout the disease course [30], repeating biopsy has also been proposed in those patients presenting with progressive disease, since it might help with planning an appropriate clinical management and therapeutic approach [31].

Additional imaging procedures were advised in the majority of patients (83.6%) after referral to the center. Interestingly, somatostatin receptor imaging (SRI) with ^{68}Ga-peptides was required in more than half of the patients (54.9%), a figure that highlights the role of this technique in the management of NEN patients. To date, SRI is considered the most effective diagnostic tool in NENs. Performing SRI may result in a change in clinical management in up to 45% of NEN patients [32], particularly due to the high ability of this technique to detect distant extra-hepatic metastases [33], whose presence is known to be a strong negative prognostic factor affecting patients' clinical outcome [34]. Changes in clinical management after multidisciplinary discussion consisted of surgical treatment in a relatively low proportion of patients (9%), although 35.4% of include patients have limited disease (Stage I–II). This figure may be due to different reasons, including the presence of patients who had been already operated on before being referred to the center, and the inclusion of patients who rarely require surgical treatment (i.e., type I gastric NENs and small rectal NENs). The present study shows that in a real-world setting of a NEN referral center, investigating tumor somatostatin receptor expression by additional SRI and advising additional histological data through the revision of available pathological data or repeating tumor biopsy are considered mandatory steps before planning patients' management. However, this study has some limitations: i. a significant proportion of patients (38.7%) were excluded from the final analysis due to the lack of relevant data, since these patients were referred to the center with the intention of obtaining a second opinion and were not followed-up; ii. the population enrolled was relatively heterogeneous, including primary tumors raising from different sites (i.e., GEP and lung); iii. The decision to request additional imaging procedures or histological evaluation was made on a case by case basis by the MDT without a specific decision-making predefined protocol; iv. data on tumor markers (i.e., Chromogranin A) were available in a minority of patients and were thus not reported in the final analysis.

5. Conclusions

A multidisciplinary approach offers the best prospect for planning optimal management and improving clinical outcomes in patients with NENs. Early referral to NEN-dedicated centers may shorten delay in diagnosis and increase the opportunity for patients to receive the best care in terms of follow-up and therapeutic approach. Enhancing referral routes to NEN-dedicated centers with experienced MDTs should be promoted, since it may improve patients' clinical outcome.

Author Contributions: Conceptualization, F.P., F.M. and M.R.; methodology, F.P., M.R.; formal analysis, L.M., G.A., F.P., and M.R.; investigation, L.M., G.A.; resources, E.P., D.P., E.I., P.P., M.R., and P.M.; data curation, F.P., F.M., and M.R.; writing—original draft preparation, F.P. and M.R.; writing—review and editing, F.P., L.M., A.S. and F.M.; visualization, all authors; supervision, A.L., A.S., P.M., and B.A.

Conflicts of Interest: The authors declare no conflict of interest.

References

1. Caplin, M.E.; Baudin, E.; Ferolla, P.; Filosso, P.; Garcia-Yuste, M.; Lim, E.; Oberg, K.; Pelosi, G.; Perren, A.; Rossi, R.E.; et al. Pulmonary neuroendocrine (carcinoid) tumors: European Neuroendocrine Tumor Society expert consensus and recommendations for best practice for typical and atypical pulmonary carcinoids. *Ann. Oncol.* **2015**, *26*, 1604–1620. [CrossRef] [PubMed]
2. Panzuto, F.; Merola, E.; Pavel, M.E.; Rinke, A.; Kump, P.; Partelli, S.; Rinzivillo, M.; Rodriguez-Laval, V.; Pape, U.F.; Lipp, R.; et al. Stage IV Gastro-Entero-Pancreatic Neuroendocrine Neoplasms: A Risk Score to Predict Clinical Outcome. *Oncologist* **2017**, *22*, 409–415. [CrossRef] [PubMed]
3. Rindi, G.; Klersy, C.; Albarello, L.; Baudin, E.; Bianchi, A.; Buchler, M.W.; Caplin, M.; Couvelard, A.; Cros, J.; de Herder, W.W.; et al. Competitive Testing of the WHO 2010 versus the WHO 2017 Grading of Pancreatic Neuroendocrine Neoplasms: Data from a Large International Cohort Study. *Neuroendocrinology* **2018**, *107*, 375–386. [CrossRef]
4. Strosberg, J. Gastroenteropancreatic Neuroendocrine Tumors. *CA Cancer J. Clin.* **2018**, *68*, 552–570.
5. Bulens, P.; Thomas, M.; Deroose, C.M.; Haustermans, K. PET imaging in adaptive radiotherapy of gastrointestinal tumors. *Q. J. Nucl. Med. Mol. Imaging* **2018**, *62*, 385–403. [CrossRef] [PubMed]
6. Opalinska, M.; Hubalewska-Dydejczyk, A.; Sowa-Staszczak, A. Radiolabeled peptides: Current and new perspectives. *Q. J. Nucl. Med. Mol. Imaging* **2017**, *61*, 153–167. [PubMed]
7. Zeelen, C.; Paus, C.; Draper, D.; Heskamp, S.; Signore, A.; Galli, F.; Griessinger, C.M.; Aarntzen., E.H. In-vivo imaging of tumor-infiltrating immune cells: Implications for cancer immunotherapy. *Q. J. Nucl. Med. Mol. Imaging* **2018**, *62*, 56–77. [PubMed]
8. Kunz, P.L.; Reidy-Lagunes, D.; Anthony, L.B.; Bertino, E.M.; Brendtro, K.; Chan, J.A.; Chen, H.; Jensen, R.T.; Kim, M.K.; Klimstra, D.S.; et al. Consensus Guidelines for the Management and Treatment of Neuroendocrine Tumors. *Pancreas* **2013**, *42*, 557–577. [CrossRef]
9. De Herder, W.W.; Capdevila, J. Unmet Needs in the Field of Neuroendocrine Neoplasms of the Gastrointestinal Tract, Pancreas, and Respiratory System: Reports by the ENETS Group. *Neuroendocrinology* **2019**, *108*, 5–6. [CrossRef]
10. Forrest, L.M.; McMillan, D.C.; McArdle, C.S.; Dunlop, D.J. An evaluation of the impact of a multidisciplinary team, in a single centre, on treatment and survival in patients with inoperable non-small-cell lung cancer. *Br. J. Cancer* **2005**, *93*, 977–978. [CrossRef]

11. Wright, F.; De Vito, C.; Langer, B.; Hunter, A. Multidisciplinary cancer conferences: A systematic review and development of practice standards. *Eur. J. Cancer* **2007**, *43*, 1002–1010. [CrossRef] [PubMed]
12. Keating, N.L.; Landrum, M.B.; Lamont, E.B.; Bozeman, S.R.; Shulman, L.N.; McNeil, B.J. Tumor Boards and the Quality of Cancer Care. *J. Natl. Cancer Inst.* **2013**, *105*, 113–121. [CrossRef] [PubMed]
13. Bosman, F.T.; Carneiro, F.; Hruban, R.H.; Theise, N.D. *WHO Classification of Tumours of the Digestive System*, 4th ed.; WHO Press: Geneva, Switzerland, 2010.
14. Lloyd, R.V.; Osamura, R.; Kloppel, G.; Rosai, J. *WHO Classification of Tumours of Endocrine Organs*, 4th ed.; IARC Press: Lyon, France, 2017.
15. Travis, W.D.; Brambilla, E.; Muller-Hermelink, H.; Harris, C.C. *Tumours of the Lung, Pleura, Thymus and Heart*; IARC Press: Lyon, France, 2004.
16. Rindi, G.; Klöppel, G.; Alhman, H.; Caplin, M.; Couvelard, A.; De Herder, W.W.; Erikssson, B.; Falchetti, A.; Falconi, M.; Komminoth, P.; et al. TNM staging of foregut (neuro)endocrine tumors: A consensus proposal including a grading system. *Virchows Archiv* **2006**, *449*, 395–401. [CrossRef] [PubMed]
17. Rindi, G.; Klöppel, G.; Couvelard, A.; Komminoth, P.; Körner, M.; Lopes, J.M.; McNicol, A.-M.; Nilsson, O.; Perren, A.; Scarpa, A.; et al. TNM staging of midgut and hindgut (neuro) endocrine tumors: A consensus proposal including a grading system. *Virchows Archiv* **2007**, *451*, 757–762. [CrossRef] [PubMed]
18. Perren, A.; Couvelard, A.; Scoazec, J.-Y.; Costa, F.; Borbath, I.; Fave, G.D.; Gorbounova, V.; Gross, D.; Grossman, A.; Jensen, R.T.; et al. ENETS Consensus Guidelines for the Standards of Care in Neuroendocrine Tumors: Pathology - Diagnosis and Prognostic Stratification. *Neuroendocrinology* **2017**, *105*, 196–200. [CrossRef]
19. Knigge, U.; Capdevila, J.; Bartsch, D.K.; Baudin, E.; Falkerby, J.; Kianmanesh, R.; Kos-Kudla, B.; Niederle, B.; Nieveen van Dijkum, E.; O'Toole, D.; et al. ENETS Consensus Recommendations for the Standards of Care in Neuroendocrine Neoplasms: Follow-Up and Documentation. *Neuroendocrinology* **2017**, *105*, 310–319. [CrossRef]
20. Metz, D.C.; Choi, J.; Strosberg, J.; Heaney, A.P.; Howden, C.W.; Klimstra, D.; Yao, J.C. A rationale for multidisciplinary care in treating neuroendocrine tumours. *Curr. Opin. Endocrinol. Diabetes Obes.* **2012**, *19*, 306–313. [CrossRef]
21. Singh, S.; Law, C. Multidisciplinary Reference Centers: The Care of Neuroendocrine Tumors. *J. Oncol. Pr.* **2010**, *6*, e11–e16. [CrossRef]
22. Fazio, N.; Ungaro, A.; Spada, F.; Cella, C.A.; Pisa, E.; Barberis, M.; Grana, C.; Zerini, D.; Bertani, E.; Ribero, D.; et al. The role of multimodal treatment in patients with advanced lung neuroendocrine tumors. *J. Thorac. Dis.* **2017**, *9*, S1501–S1510. [CrossRef]
23. Pape, U.F.; Böhmig, M.; Berndt, U.; Tiling, N.; Wiedenmann, B.; Plöckinger, U. Survival and clinical outcome of patients with neuroendocrine tumors of the gastroenteropancreatic tract in a german referral center. *Ann. N. Y. Acad. Sci.* **2004**, *1014*, 222–233. [CrossRef]
24. Panzuto, F.; Nasoni, S.; Falconi, M.; Corleto, V.D.; Capurso, G.; Cassetta, S.; Di Fonzo, M.; Tornatore, V.; Milione, M.; Angeletti, S.; et al. Prognostic factors and survival in endocrine tumor patients: Comparison between gastrointestinal and pancreatic localization. *Endocr. Relat. Cancer* **2005**, *12*, 1083–1092. [CrossRef] [PubMed]
25. Basuroy, R.; Bouvier, C.; Ramage, J.K.; Sissons, M.; Kent, A.; Srirajaskanthan, R. Presenting Symptoms and Delay in Diagnosis of Gastrointestinal and Pancreatic Neuroendocrine Tumours. *Neuroendocrinology* **2018**, *107*, 42–49. [CrossRef] [PubMed]
26. Pezzilli, R.; Partelli, S.; Cannizzaro, R.; Pagano, N.; Crippa, S.; Pagnanelli, M.; Falconi, M. Ki-67 prognostic and therapeutic decision driven marker for pancreatic neuroendocrine neoplasms (PNENs): A systematic review. *Adv. Med. Sci.* **2016**, *61*, 147–153. [CrossRef] [PubMed]
27. Lin, E.; Chen, T.; Little, A.; Holliday, L.; Roach, P.; Butler, P.; Hosking, E.; Bailey, E.; Elison, B.; Currow, D. Safety and outcomes of 177 Lu-DOTATATE for neuroendocrine tumours: Experience in New South Wales, Australia. *Intern. Med. J.* **2019**. [CrossRef] [PubMed]
28. Parghane, R.V.; Talole, S.; Basu, S. Prevalence of hitherto unknown brain meningioma detected on 68Ga-DOTATATE positron-emission tomography/computed tomography in patients with metastatic neuroendocrine tumor and exploring potential of 177Lu-DOTATATE peptide receptor radionuclide therapy as single-shot treatment approach targeting both tumors. *World J. Nucl. Med.* **2019**, *18*, 160–170. [PubMed]

29. Rindi, G.; Bordi, C.; La Rosa, S.; Solcia, E.; Fave, G.D. Gastroenteropancreatic (neuro)endocrine neoplasms: The histology report. *Dig. Liver Dis.* **2011**, *43*, S356–S360. [CrossRef]
30. Singh, S.; Hallet, J.; Rowsell, C.; Law, C. Variability of Ki67 labeling index in multiple neuroendocrine tumors specimens over the course of the disease. *Eur. J. Surg. Oncol. (EJSO)* **2014**, *40*, 1517–1522. [CrossRef]
31. Panzuto, F.; Cicchese, N.; Partelli, S.; Rinzivillo, M.; Capurso, G.; Merola, E.; Manzoni, M.; Pucci, E.; Iannicelli, E.; Pilozzi, E.; et al. Impact of Ki67 re-assessment at time of disease progression in patients with pancreatic neuroendocrine neoplasms. *PLoS ONE* **2017**, *12*, e0179445. [CrossRef]
32. Singh, S.; Poon, R.; Wong, R.; Metser, U. 68Ga PET Imaging in Patients With Neuroendocrine Tumors: A Systematic Review and Meta-analysis. *Clin. Nucl. Med.* **2018**, *43*, 802–810. [CrossRef]
33. Merola, E.; Pavel, M.E.; Panzuto, F.; Capurso, G.; Cicchese, N.; Rinke, A.; Gress, T.M.; Iannicelli, E.; Prosperi, D.; Pizzichini, P.; et al. Functional Imaging in the Follow-Up of Enteropancreatic Neuroendocrine Tumors: Clinical Usefulness and Indications. *J. Clin. Endocrinol. Metab.* **2017**, *102*, 1486–1494. [CrossRef]
34. Panzuto, F.; Merola, E.; Rinzivillo, M.; Partelli, S.; Campana, D.; Iannicelli, E.; Pilozzi, E.; Mercantini, P.; Rossi, M.; Capurso, G.; et al. Advanced digestive neuroendocrine tumors: Metastatic pattern is an independent factor affecting clinical outcome. *Pancreas* **2014**, *43*, 212–218. [CrossRef] [PubMed]

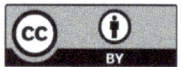

© 2019 by the authors. Licensee MDPI, Basel, Switzerland. This article is an open access article distributed under the terms and conditions of the Creative Commons Attribution (CC BY) license (http://creativecommons.org/licenses/by/4.0/).

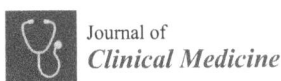

Article

Carcinoid Heart Disease and Decreased Overall Survival among Patients with Neuroendocrine Tumors: A Retrospective Multicenter Latin American Cohort Study

Deise Uema [1], Carolina Alves [2], Marcella Mesquita [2], Jose Eduardo Nuñez [2,3], Timo Siepmann [1], Martin Angel [4], Juliana F. M. Rego [5], Rui Weschenfelder [6], Duilio R. Rocha Filho [7], Frederico P. Costa [8], Milton Barros [3], Juan M. O'Connor [9], Ben M. Illigens [1,10,†] and Rachel P. Riechelmann [3,*,†]

1. Division of Health Care Sciences Center for Clinical Research and Management Education Dresden, Dresden International University, 01067 Dresden, Germany; deiseu@gmail.com (D.U.); timosiepmann.research@gmail.com (T.S.); minwootaurus@gmail.com (B.M.I.)
2. Instituto do Cancer do Estado de Sao Paulo, Sao Paulo 01246-000, Brazil; carolinaacs@hotmail.com (C.A.); cellamesquita@yahoo.com.br (M.M.); ejnunezr@gmail.com (J.E.N.)
3. Department of Clinical Oncology, AC Camargo Cancer Center, Sao Paulo 01509-900, Brazil; miltonb19@gmail.com
4. Instituto Alexander Fleming, C1426ANZ Buenos Aires, Argentina; martin.angel@hotmail.com
5. Hospital Universitário Onofre Lopes, Natal 59012-300, Brazil; juliana.oncologia@gmail.com
6. Hospital Moinhos de Vento, Porto Alegre 90035-001, Brazil; rui.fernando.w@gmail.com
7. Hospital Universitário Walter Cantídio, Fortaleza 60430-372, Brazil; duilio.rocha@uol.com.br
8. Hospital Sirio Libanês, São Paulo 01308-050, Brazil; fredericoperegocosta@gmail.com
9. Hospital de Gastroenterología Bonorino Udaondo, C1264AAA Buenos Aires, Argentina; juanmanuel.oconnor@gmail.com
10. Department of Neurology, Beth Israel Deaconess Medical Center, Harvard Medical School, Boston, MA 02114, USA
* Correspondence: Rachel.riechelmann@accamargo.org.br
† These authors contributed equally to this manuscript.

Received: 1 February 2019; Accepted: 19 March 2019; Published: 23 March 2019

Abstract: The background to this study was that factors associated with carcinoid heart disease (CHD) and its impacts on overall survival (OS) are scantly investigated in patients (pts) with neuroendocrine tumors (NETs). In terms of materials and methods, a retrospective multicenter cohort study was conducted of factors associated with CHD in advanced NET pts with carcinoid syndrome (CS) and/or elevated urinary 5-hidroxyindole acetic acid (u5HIAA). CHD was defined as at least moderate right valve alterations. The results were the following: Among the 139 subjects included, the majority had a midgut NET (54.2%), 81.3% had CS, and 93% received somatostatin analogues. In a median follow-up of 39 months, 48 (34.5%) pts developed CHD, with a higher frequency in pts treated in public (77.2%) versus private settings (22.9%). In a multivariate logistic regression, unknown primary or colorectal NETs (Odds Ratio (OR) 4.35; $p = 0.002$), at least 50% liver involvement (OR 3.45; $p = 0.005$), and being treated in public settings (OR 4.76; $p = 0.001$) were associated with CHD. In a Cox multivariate regression, bone metastases (Hazard Ratio {HR} 2.8; $p = 0.031$), CHD (HR 2.63; $p = 0.038$), and a resection of the primary tumor (HR 0.33; $p = 0.026$) influenced the risk of death. The conclusions were the following: The incidence of CHD was higher in pts with a high hepatic tumor burden and in those treated in a public system. Delayed diagnosis and limited access to effective therapies negatively affected the lives of NET patients.

Keywords: neuroendocrine tumors; carcinoid heart disease; carcinoid syndrome; somatostatin analogues; metastases

1. Introduction

Approximately 20–30% of patients with neuroendocrine tumors (NETs) are diagnosed with carcinoid syndrome (CS) in the United States [1], and it is usually associated with liver metastases and reduced overall survival [2,3]. Carcinoid syndrome, characterized by flushing, abdominal cramps, diarrhea, and bronchospasm [1,4,5], is caused by the secretion of vasoactive substances such as serotonin, histamine, prostaglandins, and tachykinins [1,5–8]. The secretion of these substances, in particular serotonin, can induce tissue fibrosis and lead to complications such as mesenteric, peritoneal, and endocardial fibrosis [8,9]. Fibrotic degeneration of the endocardium causes retraction and fixation of cardiac valves in a combination of regurgitation and stenosis, a condition known as carcinoid heart disease (CHD) [7,10]. When diagnosis is delayed, CHD can culminate with right-sided heart failure [7,10]. About 5–10% of cases have left heart involvement, and in such circumstances, lung carcinoids, patent foramen ovale, or extensive liver metastases should be suspected [11]. Because many patients with CHD do not present with symptoms until cardiopathy is in advanced stages [6,7], international guidelines recommend screening for CHD with an echocardiogram in patients with elevated urinary 5-hidroxyindole acetic acid (u5HIAA) (a metabolite of serotonin) independently of carcinoid syndrome symptoms [9,12].

The exact mechanisms causing CHD are unknown, although chronic exposure to elevated serum levels of serotonin is probably the main causal agent [13]. However, not all NET patients with elevated u5HIAA develop CHD. This observation has led to the investigation of other potential contributing factors for CHD, such as bradykinins, tachykinins, activin A, and tissue growth factor (CTGF), although no definitive marker of CHD has been defined [13]. Clinical factors associated with increased risk of CHD have also been evaluated. Retrospective studies have reported that elevated u5HIAA, the presence of flushing, and prior use of chemotherapy were significantly linked to CHD [14]. In a case-control study of 42 NET patients with elevated urinary 5-HIAA levels conducted by our group, we found that 38% developed CHD in a median follow time of 45.3 months [15]. We also observed that concurrent or prior diagnosis of a cardiovascular comorbid illness (such as coronary insufficiency or arterial hypertension) was associated with an odds ratio of 6.58 (95% confidence interval (CI) 1.09; 39.78; $p = 0.040$) for the presence of CHD. Patients with cardiovascular diseases present with endothelial dysfunction, which could predispose them to CHD in the context of other contributing factors.

Latin America lacks consistent data on cancer statistics and outcomes. Moreover, the structure of the health system, which is divided into public and private healthcare, often leads to a significant disparity in access to cancer treatment, possibly affecting recurrence and survival. While retrospective series have reported that up to 50% of patients with CS can develop carcinoid heart disease (CHD) [4,5,16], data about patients with advanced NETs and CHD in Latin America are lacking. Therefore, we conducted a multicenter study aimed at establishing a collaborative group in order to assess the incidence and risk factors for CHD as well as its impact on patients' overall survival (OS) in a Latin American cohort.

2. Material and Methods

This was a multicenter, retrospective cohort study of consecutive patients treated in eight different hospitals in Latin America (Instituto do Cancer do Estado de Sao Paulo, Sao Paulo, Brazil; Department of Oncology, AC Camargo Cancer Center, Sao Paulo, Brazil; Hospital Sirio Libanés, São Paulo, Brazil; Hospital Moinhos de Vento, Porto Alegre, Brazil; Hospital Universitário Walter Cantídio, Fortaleza, Brazil; Hospital Universitário Onofre Lopes, Natal, Brazil; Hospital de Gastroenterología Bonorino

Udaondo, Buenos Aires, Argentina; Instituto Alexander Fleming, Buenos Aires, Argentina). This study was conducted according to ICH GCP guidelines and local laws, and the protocol was submitted and approved by local Ethics Committees. The sample of this study was obtained by the evaluation of all consecutive NET cases in coparticipating hospitals: Each medical chart was reviewed for eligibility. Dubious cases were discussed with other authors so a consensus could be achieved.

All patients included were older than 18 years old, were followed between January 2000 and July 2018, had a diagnosis of advanced NETs (confirmed by biopsy), and had symptoms of carcinoid syndrome (reported as flushing, wheezing, or diarrhea, consistent with NET history) and/or elevated u5HIAA at any moment in the disease history (above the upper normal limit according to local laboratory ranges). At least one transthoracic echocardiogram (TTE) for the evaluation of CHD was required. Because of the retrospective nature of this study, a formal CHD screening protocol was not implemented in each institution. However, it is common practice among the participating centers to screen CHD every one or two years in all patients with elevated u5HIAA or CS, or when guided by symptoms. Demographics, comorbidities, tumor characteristics, oncological treatments, and information about heart conditions were collected. Due to the absence of definitive criteria for the diagnosis of CHD, it was defined in this study as at least moderate right heart valve alterations (valve thickening, reflux/regurgitation, or double lesion–stenosis and regurgitation) visualized by a TTE performed by a professional with years-long experience with CHD.

The coprimary objectives of this study were to evaluate factors that could influence the development of CHD and their impact on OS. Absolute and relative frequencies are summarized in the tables. Continuous variables were evaluated for normal distribution using both histograms and the Shapiro–Wilk test. For continuous variables with a normal distribution, the parametric unpaired Student's *t*-test was used. When the distribution was non-normal, the nonparametric Mann–Whitney *U* test was used instead. A chi-squared test was used for categorical data.

Factors potentially associated with CHD were included in univariate analysis for CHD incidence, such as gender, age, primary site (foregut (pancreas, stomach, lung), midgut, and others, which included hindgut (colorectal), others, or unknown), time from symptoms until NET diagnosis (in months), the functional status of the tumor, the extent of liver metastases (at least 50% liver involvement, which was classified by investigators based on imaging evaluation), the presence of flushing, cardiovascular comorbidities (defined as any previous or concurrent cardiovascular disease that demanded pharmacological therapy, e.g., coronary insufficiency, cerebral vascular event, or chronic high blood pressure), treatment setting (public vs private), and u5HIAA (mg/24 h) at the time of the first TTE. Variables with $p < 0.1$ were entered into a multivariable logistic regression model for CHD. In terms of factors associated with OS, besides the covariates previously mentioned, we also assessed in a univariate Cox proportional-hazards model the following covariates: The presence of CHD, resection of the primary tumor, and bone metastasis. Covariates deemed as significant ($p < 0.1$) in a univariate regression were then entered into the multivariate Cox proportional-hazards model. For OS, the multivariate stepwise model, which sequentially removes each covariate at a time, was applied until the best OS model was found.

All statistical tests were two-sided, with the α level set at 0.05. A Strobe checklist was used to ensure the completeness of the information reported in this retrospective study [17]. All analyses were performed in the whole study population, as patients with significant missing data were excluded (see "Results", Figure 1).

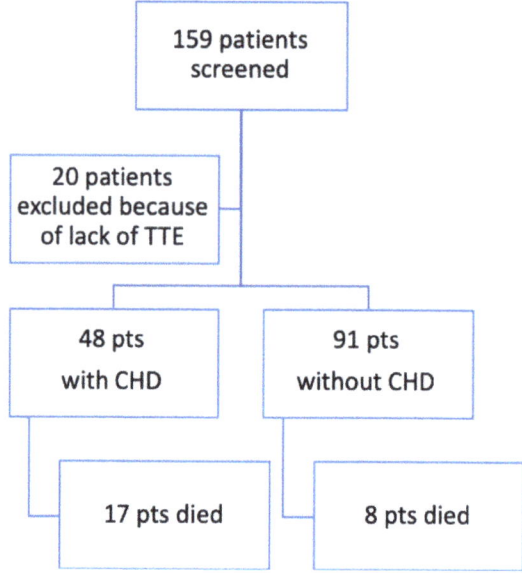

Figure 1. Flowchart of patient selection and inclusion.

3. Results

One-hundred and fifty-nine patients with advanced disease and carcinoid symptoms and/or elevated u5HIAA were identified in the electronic health records of the participating hospitals. Of these, 139 were eligible and were included in the analysis herein conducted (see flow diagram below).

For CHD incidence, all 139 patients had complete data, while for the OS evaluation, 127 patients out of 139 had all selected factors complete and were included in the analysis. With a median follow-up time of 39 months (range: 2.7–150.6 months), 48 patients (34.5%) developed CHD, and 91 patients (65.5%) remained CHD-free.

The baseline demographic characteristics of the whole population and subgroups based on CHD occurrence are described in Table 1.

Among all patients, midgut tumors were the most common primary site, 81.3% had CS, and 93% received somatostatin analogues.

The mean age at diagnosis of an NET was 56.52 years (±14.8 years) in patients with CHD compared to 51.9 years (±12.54 years) in patients without CHD ($p = 0.049$). Both groups had a similar median time from the beginning of symptoms until diagnosis of an NET (CHD 10.93 months vs non-CHD 9.03 months; $p = 0.285$). A significantly higher proportion of patients with CHD had NETs of other origins, such as colorectal and unknown primary sites (CHD 35.4% vs. non-CHD 11%; $p = 0.001$).

Other factors significantly more frequently encountered among CHD patients were at least 50% of liver volume involved by metastases (CHD 41.7% vs. non-CHD 23.1%; $p = 0.037$), median u5HIAA (mg/24 h) at the time of the first TTE (CHD 40 mg/24 h vs. 18.1 mg/24 h non-CHD ($p = 0.05$)), the proportion of patients treated in a public setting (CHD: Public setting 77.1% vs private setting 22.9%; $p = 0.001$).

Table 1. Baseline demographic characteristics of the study population.

		With Carcinoid Heart Disease		Without Carcinoid Heart Disease		Whole Population		p-Value **
		No. of Subjects	%	No. of Subjects	%	No. of Subjects	%	
Gender	Female	27	56.3	47	52.2	74	53.2	0.735 *
	Male	21	43.7	44	47.8	65	46.8	
Age at diagnosis (years)	Mean ± SD	56.52 ± 14.8		51.9 ± 12.5		53.5 ± 13.5		0.049 #
Time from beginning of symptoms until diagnosis of an NET (months)	Median (range)	10.93 (0–107.9)		7.17 (0–160.6)		9.03 (0–160.6)		0.285
Grouped primary site	Foregut (pancreas/stomach)	5	10.4	13	14.3	18	13.0	0.001 *
	Midgut	26	54.2	68	74.7	94	67.6	
	Colorectal, unknown primary, others	17	35.4	10	11.0	27	19.4	
Staging	Metastatic	45	93.75	78	85.71	123	88.49	
WHO Classification	Grade 1	24	50	34	37.36	58	41.73	
	Grade 2	16	33.33	33	36.26	49	35.25	
	Grade 3	2	4.17	1	1.1	3	2.16	
Median Ki67-% (Range)		2.2 (1–60)		2.0 (1–25)		2.0 (1–60)		
Differentiation	Well differentiated	42	87.5	82	90.11	124	89.21	
Functional status	Functioning	42	87.5	71	78.0	113	81.3	0.257 *
Flushing	Yes	31	64.6	48	52.7	79	56.8	0.246 *
Liver metastases	At least 50% involvement	20	41.7	21	23.1	41	29.5	
Bone metastases	Yes	8	16.7	11	12.09	19	13.67	
Cardiovascular comorbidities	Yes	20	41.7	40	44.0	60	43.2	0.937 *
Treatment setting	Public	37	77.1	42	46.2	79	56.8	0.001 *
	Private	11	22.9	49	53.8	60	43.2	
Resection of primary tumor	Yes	24	51.0	61	67.0	85	61.6	
Metastasectomy	Yes	14	29.2	33	36.3	47	33.8	
u5HIAA (mg/24 h) at 1st TTE	Median (Range)	40 (5.4–271.2)		18.1 (2.8–22365)		23.7 (2.8–22365)		0.05 ##

** p-value presented for comparison of covariates between patients with carcinoid heart disease (CHD) and without CHD; * chi-squared test; # parametric Student's t-test; ## nonparametric Mann–Whitney U test; SD = standard deviation; NET = neuroendocrine tumor; u5HIAA = urinary 5-hydroxyindole-3-acetic acid; TTE = transthoracic echocardiogram.

Univariate and multivariate logistic regression models showed that primary site, extent of liver metastases, and treatment setting were predictive ($p < 0.05$) for the occurrence of CHD. In multivariate analysis, while holding the two other covariates constant, the odds of presenting with CHD with a primary site of "others" (colorectal, unknown primary, and others such as ovary, peritoneum, lung, etc.) were 4.35 times the odds of presenting with CHD for tumors from the pancreas/stomach or midgut ($p = 0.002$). Similarly, the odds of presenting with CHD with metastases involving more than 50% of liver volume were 3.45 times the odds of presenting with CHD in the group with lower metastatic liver involvement ($p = 0.005$). The odds of presenting with CHD in patients treated in a public setting were 4.76 times the odds of presenting with this condition in patients treated in a private setting ($p = 0.001$), as shown in Table 2.

Table 2. Results of univariate and multivariate analyses for CHD incidence. CI: Confidence interval; OR: Odds Ratio.

Covariates	Univariate OR (CI 95%)	Univariate p-Value	Multivariate OR (CI 95%)	Multivariate p-Value
Age at diagnosis	1.03 (1.00; 1.05)	0.057		
Gender Female	1.20 (0.60; 2.43)	0.605		
Primary site Hindgut, unknown primary, or others	2.63 (1.72; 4.00)	<0.001	4.35 (1.67; 11.11)	0.002
Time from symptoms until NET diagnosis (months)	1.00 (0.99; 1.02)	0.616		
Functioning tumor	1.97 (0.73; 5.30)	0.178		
More than 50% liver involvement	2.5 (1.61; 3.85)	<0.001	3.45 (1.47; 8.33)	0.005
Treatment in public setting	4.55 (2.33; 8.33)	<0.001	4.76 (1.92; 11.11)	0.001
Presence of flushing	1.63 (0.79; 3.36)	0.182		
Cardiovascular comorbidities	0.91 (0.45; 1.85)	0.796		
u5HIAA at 1st TTE	1 (0.999; 1)	0.657		

In terms of OS, the univariate Cox regression showed that age at NET diagnosis, primary site of tumor, occurrence of CHD, resection of primary tumor, setting of treatment (public vs. private), and bone metastases were significantly associated with OS.

In the Cox multivariate regression stepwise model, CHD (HR 2.63, $p = 0.038$), resection of primary NET (HR: 0.33, $p = 0.026$), and bone metastases (HR = 2.8, $p = 0.031$) independently influenced the risk of death, as shown in Table 3.

As shown in Table 4, the most frequently affected heart valve in patients with CHD was the tricuspid valve (50%), followed by a compromise of the tricuspid and pulmonary valves (27.08%) and, to a lesser extent, both right and left heart valves (20.83%). The most common alterations were valve insufficiency (45.8%) and a combination of valve thickening and insufficiency (45.8%). Isolated valve thickening or stenosis was uncommon (20.8%). In terms of severity, the majority of patients had severe alterations in TTEs (31.30%) or severe alterations with dilations of heart chambers or decreased ejection fraction (50%) at the moment of CHD diagnosis. In this sample, only two patients with CHD had corrective valvuloplasty or surgery.

Table 3. Results of univariate Cox regression and multi-Cox regression for overall survival (OS).

Covariates	Univariate OR (CI 95%)	Univariate p-Value	Multivariate * OR (CI95%)	Multivariate * p-Value
Age at diagnosis	1.06 (1.02; 1.11)	0.001	1.05 (1.00; 1.09)	0.028
Gender Female	1.78 (0.75; 4.26)	0.193		
Primary site Hindgut, unknown primary, or others	2.70 (1.12; 6.67)	0.026		
CHD	3.75 (1.53; 9.20)	0.004	2.63 (1.05; 6.56)	0.038
Primary tumor resection	0.27 (0.11; 0.65)	0.004	0.33 (0.13; 0.87)	0.026
Functioning tumor	3.51 (0.47; 26.16)	0.221		
More than 50% liver involvement	1.28 (0.58; 3.03)	0.579		
Treatment in public setting	4.00 (1.22; 11.11)	0.013		
Bone metastases	2.7 (1.10; 6.62)	0.030	2.80 (1.10; 7.13)	0.031

* Multivariate stepwise model.

Table 4. Echocardiographic alterations in patients with CHD.

	N	%
Heart valves affected		
Tricuspid	24	50.00
Tricuspid and pulmonary	13	27.08
Right and left heart	10	20.83
Type of alteration	N	%
Valve thickening	1	2.08
Valve insufficiency	22	45.80
Thickening and insufficiency	22	45.80
Stenosis	2	4.17
Severity	N	%
Mild	2	4.17
Moderate	7	14.60
Severe	15	31.30
Severe with dilation or decreased ejection fraction	24	50.00

In a median follow-up of 39 months, the median overall survival of patients with CHD was not reached because of the number of events censored. Of the 47 patients with a survival time after CHD diagnosis (time of CHD–months) available, only 17 patients (36.2%) died, while the other 30 patients (63.8%) were still alive at the time of data collection for this study: The mean OS was 68.89 months (95% CI: 50.47–83.32).

After a CHD diagnosis, the OS rate at 1 year was 79%, and at 5 years it was 54%.

Given the strong association between CHD and OS with treatment delivered in the public system, we present in Table 5 the summarized characteristics of patients according to treatment setting. Patients treated in a public setting had a longer time from the beginning of symptoms until a diagnosis of NET, had a higher incidence of CHD, and had more cardiovascular comorbid illnesses. In addition, primary tumors were resected less frequently, and they were less exposed to more than one line of systemic therapy.

Table 5. Summarized characteristics of patients according to treatment setting (pts = patients).

Covariates	Public	Private
Median age at diagnosis	58 years	49 years
Time from beginning of symptoms until NET diagnosis	12 months	6.7 months
CHD	46.8% (37/79 pts)	18.3% (11/60 pts)
More than 50% liver involvement	25.3% (20/79 pts)	35% (21/60 pts)
Cardiovascular comorbid illnesses	48.1% (38/79 pts)	36.6% (22/60 pts)
Primary tumor resected	54.4% (43/79 pts)	70% (42/60 pts)
Bone metastases	8.8% (7/79 pts)	20% (12/60 pts)
Flushing	65.8% (52/79 pts)	45% (27/60 pts)
Carcinoid syndrome	87.3% (69/79 pts)	73.3% (44/60 pts)
Somatostatin analogues use	91.1% (72/79 pts)	95% (57/60 pts)
Received more than one systemic treatment	27.8% (22/79 pts)	60% (36/60 pts)

4. Discussion

In this multicenter retrospective cohort study, the largest conducted in Latin America and among the largest series of CHD cases worldwide, we evaluated the incidence of CHD and the impact on OS of patients with advanced NETs, in addition to the already known adverse prognostic factors. We observed that nearly one-third of patients developed CHD in a median follow-up of 39 months. Factors independently associated with CHD were treatment delivered in a public setting, unknown primary or colorectal NET, and at least 50% liver involvement by metastases. In addition, u5HIAA levels were higher among CHD patients. CHD and bone metastases increased the risk of death, and resection of the primary tumor was a protective factor from mortality.

We found that patients with a larger burden of liver metastases (≥50% of liver volume affected) were more likely to present with CHD [10,11]. CHD is thought to be caused by the action of vasoactive substances in the endocardium [14]. Therefore, it is reasonable to expect that when the production of vasoactive substances exceeds liver metabolism, a larger amount of these substances will reach the right heart, increasing the chances of CHD development [2,6,10,11]. It is believed that some tumors, such as primary NETs in bronchi, ovaries, testes, lymph nodes, and the retroperitoneum, have direct access to systemic circulation, and in this subgroup, CHD frequently occurs in the absence of liver metastases or carcinoid syndrome symptoms [2,3,6,10].

Serotonin seems to play an important role in CHD development, as it induces tissue fibrosis [10,18]. In agreement with previous research, our study showed that urinary serotonin metabolite 5HIAA levels were significantly higher in patients with CHD compared to patients without CHD, supporting the value of u5HIAA as a screening tool for CHD [14,18]. Considering the importance of the hepatic metabolization and location of the primary tumor, it is not surprising that in some studies, u5HIAA has been more precise in predicting the progression of CHD than the radiological progression of the tumor burden [18]. The positive association between cardiovascular comorbidities and CHD observed in our prior study [15] was not found in the present study with a larger sample size. It is possible that the finding from our previous study was a false positive: However, we think that future studies should evaluate cardiovascular comorbid illnesses as a potential risk factor for CHD.

On our opinion, the most important and original result of our study was the significant association between CHD and treatment in a public setting. This likely reflects delayed access or lack of access to effective systemic anticancer therapies and suboptimal supportive care. Therefore, our data strongly suggests that treating carcinoid symptoms, i.e., decreasing exposure to elevated levels of serotonin, prevents or delays CHD. As shown in Table 5, patients in a public setting had a longer interval from the beginning of symptoms until diagnosis of an NET, had lower rates of primary tumor resection, and were less frequently exposed to more than one systemic therapy. The diagnosis of NETs requires a high level of suspicion because of its relative rarity and generic symptoms. Therefore, with a scarcity of ancillary tests, these "indolent tumors" may progress undetected for a prolonged period, leading to a delayed diagnosis. Once the diagnosis is made, NET optimal treatment needs the coordinated action of a multidisciplinary team to ensure the best outcome. In addition to these challenges, in our public healthcare setting, several patients still need to obtain somatostatin analogues via judicialization, as it is not made available in all public services, which delays even further the systemic treatment of metastatic disease. These findings possibly corroborate the prognostic factor "year of diagnosis" found in the Surveillance, Epidemiology and End Results program registry [19]. Having chosen the year of octreotide introduction to the United States (1987), Yao et al. were able to show a positive shift in the survival curve, demonstrating the relevance of the inclusion of somatostatin analogues and enhanced supportive treatment for patients with advanced NETs [16,19,20]. A lack of CHD screening and inappropriate management also seem to play a significant role in the observed higher incidence of CHD in the public system and the related shortened survival.

In our study, CHD was a prognostic factor for mortality, although median survival was not reached due to the low number of events in the median follow-up time of 39 months. Considering that in 1993, Pellikka et al. reported a median overall survival of 1.6 years for CHD patients [4], our median follow-up time seemed appropriate for estimating the median survival of our CHD group. More recent series, such as the study reported by Connolly et al., have reported a 69% OS at 1 year and a 34% OS at 5 years [16], while in our study, the OS rates were 79% at 1 year and 54% at 5 years. These differences in OS rates and median survivals likely reflected our definition of CHD, which considered patients with moderate and severe valve alterations in comparison to other studies that may have included patients with more severe heart valve dysfunctions who were being considered for valve replacements [16]. In addition, a longer follow-up would have been necessary to properly evaluate the OS in our sample [21].

Unfortunately, in contrast to the current evidence that suggests that valve surgery may improve mortality in patients with symptomatic severe right heart valve disease [16,20], only two patients in our sample underwent cardiac surgery, despite more than 80% presenting with severe valve dysfunction as detected by TTE. This likely reflects the poor access to cardiac surgery among patients treated in the public systems of Latin America.

Resection of the primary tumor has also been associated with increased OS and is likely related to a reduction in vasoactive substance production [18] and potentially fatal complications such as bowel obstruction. An alternative explanation for tumor resection and improved OS could be the fact that patients who undergo surgical resection may have a lower metastatic tumor burden and are thus amenable to surgical resection.

The limitations of our study should be pointed out. The retrospective nature of our study may have limited the validity of our findings. We could not evaluate other prognostic markers, such as pro-pro-brain natriuretic peptide, response to treatment, patterns of radiological progression, or even tissue tumor biomarkers, which could have provided us with a deeper understanding of the mechanisms that lead to the development of CHD. The intervals of TTE were not standardized, and this may have underestimated the true incidence of CHD because of the number of patients who were asymptomatic and did not have a recent TTE: TTEs were performed annually or biannually.

Although the use of complete case analysis may have favored the observation of patients with better (or worse) prognostic features, the amount of missing data was below 10%. Nonetheless, considering that this was a multicentric study and the largest conducted in a Latin American population, these findings certainly establish the feasibility of such an effort and provide us some guidance for future collaborative prospective studies. It also brings awareness to the alarmingly high incidence of CHD in patients treated in our public systems. Governments should devote more resources to treating NET patients, particularly those with functioning tumors.

In conclusion, in order to diagnose CHD in a timely manner, clinicians should be attentive and aware of the risk of patients with advanced NETs developing such a complication. Our study reinforces the recommendation of performing annual TTEs for patients with elevated u5HIAA. For patients with a low hepatic tumor burden or for those with a primary tumor in the foregut or midgut, screening TTE frequency can possibly be reduced, while for patients with a high hepatic tumor burden and tumors in the hindgut or other locations, as well as those with delayed access or lack of access to antitumor therapies, annual screenings should be strictly maintained or performed even more frequently. Treatment in a public setting was associated with higher chances of developing CHD, underlining the negative impact that disparities in access to healthcare have in terms of cancer outcomes. This highlights the adverse effect of delayed diagnosis and treatment and emphasizes the importance of appropriate CHD screening and early treatment of patients with elevated u5HIAA to offer the best survival chances for patients with advanced NETs.

Author Contributions: Conceptualization, R.P.R.; methodology: D.U., R.P.R; validation, D.U., R.P.R., R.W., J.M.O.C., J.E.N., M.M., C.A., M.B., B.M.I; formal analysis, D.U., R.P.R., B.M.I., T.S.; resources, D.U., R.P.R., R.W., J.M.O.C, J.E.N, M.M, C.A, F.P.C., M.A., J.F.M.R., D.R.R.F., B.M.I, T.S, M.B.; data curation, D.U., R.P.R., R.W., J.M.O.C., J.E.N., M.M., C.A, F.P.C, J.F.M.R, D.R.R.F, writing—original draft preparation, D.U., R.P.R. writing—review and editing, D.U., R.P.R., R.W., J.M.O.C, J.E.N., M.M., C.A, F.P.C, M.A., J.F.M.R., D.R.R.F., B.M.I, T.S, M.B.; visualization, D.U., R.P.R., R.W., J.M.O.C, J.E.N., M.M., C.A, F.P.C, M.A., J.F.M.R., D.R.R.F., B.M.I, T.S, M.B.; supervision, R.P.R.; project administration, R.P.R.

Funding: The author J.E.N was funded through a Neuroendocrine Fellowship Program by the Brazilian Society of Clinical Oncology (SBOC).

Acknowledgments: This work is part of a Master's thesis of the Master's Program in Clinical Research, Center for Clinical Research and Management Education, Division of Health Care Sciences, Dresden International University, Dresden, Germany.

Conflicts of Interest: R.P.R. has received consultancy and research grants from Ipsen; R.P.R., D.R.R.F., R.W., J.F.M.R., J.M.O.C., M.B. have received honoraria from Novartis and Ipsen.

References

1. Raja, S.G.; Bhattacharyya, S.; Davar, J.; Dreyfus, G.D. Surgery for carcinoid heart disease: Current outcomes, concerns and controversies. *Future Cardiol.* **2010**, *6*, 647–655. [CrossRef] [PubMed]
2. Feldman, J.M.; Jones, R.S. Carcinoid Syndrome from Gastrointestinal Carcinoids without Liver Metastasis. *Ann Surg* **1982**, *196*, 33. [CrossRef] [PubMed]
3. Haq, A.U.; Yook, C.R.; Hiremath, V.; Kasimis, B.S. Carcinoid Syndrome in the Absence of Liver Metastasis: A Case Report and Review of Literature. *Med. Pediatr. Oncol.* **1992**, *20*, 221–223. [CrossRef] [PubMed]
4. Pellikka, P.A.; Tajik, A.J.; Khandheria, B.K.; Seward, J.B.; Callahan, J.A.; Pitot, H.C.; Kvols, L.K. Carcinoid heart disease. Clinical and echocardiographic spectrum in 74 patients. *Circulation* **1993**, *87*, 1188–1196. [CrossRef] [PubMed]
5. Connolly, H.M.; Schaff, H.V.; Mullany, C.J.; Rubin, J.; Abel, M.D.; Pellikka, P.A. Surgical Management of Left-Sided Carcinoid Heart Disease. *Circulation* **2001**, *104* (Suppl. 1), I36–I40. [CrossRef]
6. Grozinsky-Glasberg, S.; Grossman, A.B.; Gross, D.J. Carcinoid Heart Disease: From Pathophysiology to Treatment—"Something in the Way It Moves". *Neuroendocrinology* **2015**, *101*, 263–273. [CrossRef] [PubMed]
7. Dobson, R.; Burgess, M.I.; Pritchard, D.M.; Cuthbertson, D.J. The clinical presentation and management of carcinoid heart disease. *Int. J. Cardiol.* **2014**, *173*, 29–32. [CrossRef] [PubMed]
8. Mota, J.M.; Sousa, L.G.; Riechelmann, R.P. Complications from carcinoid syndrome: Review of the current evidence. *Ecancermedicalscience* **2016**, *10*, 662. [CrossRef] [PubMed]

9. Pape, U.-F.; Perren, A.; Niederle, B.; Gross, D.; Gress, T.; Costa, F.; Arnold, R.; Denecke, T.; Plöckinger, U.; Salazar, R.; et al. ENETS Consensus Guidelines for the Management of Patients with Neuroendocrine Neoplasms from the Jejuno-Ileum and the Appendix Including Goblet Cell Carcinomas. *Neuroendocrinology* **2012**, *95*, 135–156. [CrossRef]
10. Gustafsson, B.I.; Hauso, O.; Drozdov, I.; Kidd, M.; Modlin, I.M. Carcinoid heart disease. *Int. J. Cardiol.* **2008**, *129*, 318–324. [CrossRef] [PubMed]
11. Fox, D.J.; Khattar, R.S. Carcinoid Heart Disease: Presentation, Diagnosis, and Management. *Heart* **2004**, *90*, 1224–1228. [CrossRef] [PubMed]
12. Riechelmann, R.P.; Weschenfelder, R.F.; Costa, F.P.; Chaves Andrade, A.; Bersch Osvald, A.; Quidute, A.R.P.; Dos Santos, A.; Hoff, A.A.O.; Gumz, B.; Buchpiguel, C.; et al. Guidelines for the management of neuroendocrine tumours by the Brazilian gastrointestinal tumour group. *Ecancermedicalscience* **2017**, *11*, 716. [CrossRef] [PubMed]
13. Ferrari, A.; Glasberg, J.; Riechelmann, R. Carcinoid syndrome: Update on the pathophysiology and treatment. *Clinics* **2018**, *73* (Suppl. 1), e490s. [CrossRef]
14. Møller, J.E.; Connolly, H.M.; Rubin, J.; Seward, J.B.; Modesto, K.; Pellikka, P.A. Factors Associated with Progression of Carcinoid Heart Disease. *N. Engl. J. Med.* **2003**, *348*, 1005–1015. [CrossRef]
15. Alves, C.; Mesquita, M.; Silva, C.; Soeiro, M.; Hajjar, L.; Riechelmann, R.P. High tumour burden, delayed diagnosis and history of cardiovascular disease may be associated with carcinoid heart disease. *Ecancermedicalscience* **2018**, *12*, 879. [CrossRef] [PubMed]
16. Connolly, H.M.; Schaff, H.V.; Abel, M.D.; Rubin, J.; Askew, J.W.; Li, Z.; Inda, J.J.; Luis, S.A.; Nishimura, R.A.; Pellikka, P.A. Early and late outcomes of surgical treatment in carcinoid heart disease. *J. Am. Coll. Cardiol.* **2015**. [CrossRef]
17. STROBE. STROBE 2007 (v4) Statement—Checklist of items that should be included in reports of cohort studies. *PLoS Med.* **2007**. Available online: https://bmjopen.bmj.com/content/suppl/2012/01/06/bmjopen-2011-000186.DC1/STROBE_checklist.pdf (accessed on 20 March 2019).
18. Dobson, R.; Burgess, M.I.; Valle, J.W.; Pritchard, D.M.; Vora, J.; Wong, C.; Chadwick, C.; Keevi, B.; Adaway, J.; Hofmann, U.; et al. Serial surveillance of carcinoid heart disease: Factors associated with echocardiographic progression and mortality. *Br. J. Cancer* **2014**, *111*, 1703. [CrossRef]
19. Yao, J.C.; Hassan, M.; Phan, A.; Dagohoy, C.; Leary, C.; Mares, J.E.; Abdalla, E.K.; Fleming, J.B.; Vauthey, J.N.; Rashid, A.; et al. One hundred years after "carcinoid": Epidemiology of and prognostic factors for neuroendocrine tumors in 35,825 cases in the United States. *J. Clin. Oncol.* **2008**, *26*, 3063–3072. [CrossRef]
20. Warner, R.R.P.; Castillo, J.G. Carcinoid heart disease: The challenge of the unknown known. *J. Am. Coll. Cardiol.* **2015**. [CrossRef] [PubMed]
21. Westberg, G.; Wängberg, B.; Ahlman, H.; Bergh, C.H.; Beckman-Suurküla, M.; Caidahl, K. Prediction of prognosis by echocardiography in patients with midgut carcinoid syndrome. *Br. J. Surg.* **2001**. [CrossRef] [PubMed]

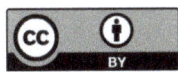

© 2019 by the authors. Licensee MDPI, Basel, Switzerland. This article is an open access article distributed under the terms and conditions of the Creative Commons Attribution (CC BY) license (http://creativecommons.org/licenses/by/4.0/).

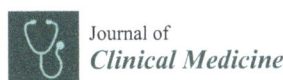

Article

Treatment of Liver Metastases from Midgut Neuroendocrine Tumours: A Systematic Review and Meta-Analysis

Enes Kaçmaz [1], Charlotte M. Heidsma [1], Marc G. H. Besselink [1], Koen M. A. Dreijerink [2], Heinz-Josef Klümpen [3,4,5], Elisabeth J. M. Nieveen van Dijkum [1,4] and Anton F. Engelsman [1,4,*]

1. Department of Surgery, Amsterdam UMC, University of Amsterdam, Meibergdreef 9, 1105 AZ Amsterdam, The Netherlands; e.kacmaz@amc.uva.nl (E.K.); c.m.heidsma@amc.uva.nl (C.M.H.); m.g.besselink@amc.uva.nl (M.G.H.B.); e.j.nieveenvandijkum@amc.uva.nl (E.J.M.N.v.D.)
2. Department of Endocrinology, Amsterdam UMC, Vrije Universiteit Amsterdam, 1081 HV Amsterdam, The Netherlands; k.dreijerink@vumc.nl
3. Department of Oncology, Amsterdam UMC, University of Amsterdam, 1105 AZ Amsterdam, The Netherlands; h.klumpen@amc.uva.nl
4. ENETS Center of Excellence, Amsterdam UMC, University of Amsterdam, 1105 AZ Amsterdam, The Netherlands
5. Cancer Center Amsterdam, 1182 DB Amsterdam, The Netherlands
* Correspondence: a.f.engelsman@amc.uva.nl

Received: 20 February 2019; Accepted: 18 March 2019; Published: 22 March 2019

Abstract: Strong evidence comparing different treatment options for liver metastases (LM) arising from gastroenteropancreatic neuroendocrine tumours (GEP-NET) is lacking. The aim of this study was to determine which intervention for LMs from GEP-NETs shows the longest overall survival (OS). A systematic search was performed in MEDLINE, Embase and the Cochrane Library in February 2018. Studies reporting on patients with LMs of any grade of sporadic GEP-NET comparing two intervention groups were included for analysis. Meta-analyses were performed where possible. Eleven studies, with a total of 1108, patients were included; 662 patients had LM from pancreatic NETs (pNET), 164 patients from small-bowel NETs (SB-NET) and 282 patients of unknown origin. Improved 5-year OS was observed for surgery vs. chemotherapy (OR 0.05 95% CI [0.01, 0.21] $p < 0.0001$), for surgery vs. embolization (OR 0.18 95% CI [0.05, 0.61] $p = 0.006$) and for LM resection vs. no LM resection (OR 0.15 95% CI [0.05, 0.42] $p = 0.0003$). This is the largest meta-analysis performed comparing different interventions for LMs from GEP-NETs. Despite the high risk of bias and heterogeneity of data, surgical resection for all tumour grades results in the longest overall survival. Chemotherapy and embolization should be considered as an alternative in case surgery is not feasible.

Keywords: small bowel neuroendocrine tumours; pancreatic neuroendocrine tumours; liver metastases; midgut; meta-analysis

1. Introduction

Gastroenteropancreatic neuroendocrine tumours (GEP-NET) represent a heterogeneous group of tumours arising from neuroendocrine cells of the gastro-intestinal tract. The annual incidence of GEP-NETs is estimated to be around 2.88 (European standardized rate, ESR) [1]. In specialized centres, liver metastases (LM) are diagnosed in up to 80–90% of patients with small-bowel NETs (SB-NET) and 60–70% of patients with pancreatic neuroendocrine NETs (pNET) [2]. LM is the strongest predictor for poor survival of patients with GEP-NET regardless of the location of the primary tumour with a 5-year overall survival of 13–54 months for patients with untreated LM [3].

Treatment of patients with LM is aimed at local tumour control and symptom relief. Several treatment modalities for NET-LMs exist, and include resection or debulking of the metastases, radiofrequency ablation (RFA), tumour embolization and pharmacological treatment. Pharmacologic interventions include somatostatin analogues (SSA), targeted therapy, peptide receptor radionuclide therapy (PRRT), chemotherapy and immunotherapy. SSAs reduce hormone associated symptoms in patients, while lengthening progression free survival (PFS) [4–6]. The phase 3 NETTER-trial showed improvement in PFS when treating patients with 177-Lu-Dotatate (PRRT) and octreotide with long acting release (LAR) versus octreotide LAR alone in patients with well differentiated metastatic midgut NETs [7]. The protein kinase inhibitor everolimus and sunitinib also increase PFS in patients with advanced NETs [8–10]. Hepatic artery embolization (HAE) prolongs survival, whilst being safe and feasible [11]. Current ENETS guidelines state that SSA, octreotide and lanreotide are equally effective in both symptom control and antiproliferative effect [12].

A systematic review published in 2008 by Gurusamy et al. aimed to compare liver resection to other treatment modalities in patients with LMs from GEP-NETs, but were unable to conduct an analysis due to a lack of relevant articles at that time [13]. In the past decade, multiple cohort studies were published. The aim of this systematic review is to determine which treatment modality leads to highest overall survival in patients with LM from GEP-NETs.

2. Methods

2.1. Search Strategy

A systematic search was performed in MEDLINE (PubMed), Embase (Ovid) and the Cochrane Library on 1 February 2018 (Supplementary Material S1). The search strategy is presented in Supplementary Material S1 and included both keywords and MeSH terms: 'neuroendocrine tumours', 'midgut', 'liver metastasis', 'pancreatic neoplasms', 'duodenal neoplasms', 'ileal neoplasms', 'jejunal neoplasms', 'somatostatin', 'interferons', 'molecular targeted therapy', 'chemotherapy', 'surgery', 'surgical oncology', and 'catheter ablation'. No publication date restriction was used. Studies published in any language other than English were excluded. This study was registered in PROSPERO with the following registration number: CRD42018104328.

2.2. In- and Exclusion Criteria

All randomized controlled trials, cross-sectional, cohort studies and case-series reporting on treatment of GEP-NET related LM with at least 5 patients in a minimum of two compared intervention groups were eligible for inclusion. All grades of GEP-NETs were included. Patients with mixed neuroendocrine or non-neuroendocrine neoplasms (MINEN/MENEN) were excluded. No age limit was applied.

2.3. Study Selection

All studies identified by the search were screened for eligibility by two independent authors (AE, EK) using Rayyan software (Qatar Computing Research Institute, Doha, Qatar) [14]. After selection based on title and abstract, full texts were analysed for further in- or exclusion. Any conflicts arising from the selection were resolved by consensus. The 5-year overall survival or 5-year disease specific survival after intervention had to be stated in the study, or the data to calculate this had to be available. No strict definition of a curative or palliative resection had to be met. Patients with LM from pancreatic, duodenal, jejunal or ileal NETs were included. In case of publications with overlapping patient cohorts, the study with the largest cohort size was included for analysis.

2.4. Data Extraction

The following characteristics were extracted: patient characteristics, primary tumour location (pancreas or small bowel), type of therapy for LM, resection of the primary tumour, LM status (resectable/unresectable), uni- or bilobar metastases, extrahepatic disease, WHO (World Health Organization) 2010 grade and follow-up period. The primary outcome was 5-year overall survival. Secondary outcomes included disease free survival (DFS), progression free survival (PFS) and post-operative complications. Subgroups for analysis were defined as resection of primary tumour versus no resection at all, LM resection versus no resection at all, any resection versus chemotherapy, any resection versus embolization and any resection versus LTx (liver transplantation). 'No resection at all' was defined as no LM nor primary resection, 'any resection' was defined as a primary with or without LM resection.

2.5. Statistical Analysis

For the meta-analysis, outcome data stratified by subgroups were pooled using Review Manager 5.3 (The Nordic Cochrane Centre, The Cochrane Collaboration, Denmark, Copenhagen) and presented in a forest plot. Heterogeneity was assessed by calculating the I^2 index. An $I^2 < 25\%$ was considered as low and a fixed effects model was used for the meta-analysis using and the Mantel–Haenszel method [15]. An I^2 between 25–75% was considered as intermediate and consequently a random effects model was used for the meta-analysis. An $I^2 > 75\%$ was considered substantial and no meta-analysis was performed. Funnel plots were made to assess publication bias.

2.6. Risk of Bias Assessment

The ROBINS-I (Risk of Bias in Non-randomized Studies—of Intervention) tool was used to assess risk of bias for the included studies [16].

3. Results

3.1. Description of Studies

A total of 712 studies were identified through the electronic search in MEDLINE (PubMed), Embase and the Cochrane Library. After the screening and selection process, 11 studies fulfilled the inclusion criteria (Figure 1) [17–27]. Characteristics of the included studies are presented in Table 1. There were no randomized controlled trials found. The 11 included studies represent a total of 1108 patients, of which 662 patients had pNETs, 164 patients had SB-NETs and 282 patients had a tumour originating from lungs ($n = 26$), ovaries ($n = 1$) and unknown primary locations ($n = 102$) (Table 2). Out of all included studies, five intervention groups were composed: primary tumour resection versus no resection at all, LM resection versus no resection at all, any resection versus chemotherapy, any resection versus embolization and any resection versus LTx.

Table 1. Characteristics of included studies.

Author	Country	Design	No. Patients (n)	Inclusion Criteria Per Study	Exclusion Criteria Per Study	Intervention Groups	Control Group
Watzka et al. [27]	DE	Retrospective	204	Patients with LM of NEN.	N/A	Radical LM resection (n = 38)	No resection at all (n = 110)
Partelli et al. [26]	IT	Retrospective	166	Patients with synchronous LM from sporadic pNET.	Patients with extra-abdominal disease as well as those with peritoneal carcinomatosis and those with an inherited syndrome.	Radical LM resection + primary resection (n = 18)	No resection at all (n = 75) (SSA; PRRT; chemotherapy; everolimus or sunitinib)
Citterio et al. [21]	IT	Retrospective	139	≤20 mitoses/10 high power field (HPF) and Ki-67 labelling index ≤ 20% at either the primary or metastatic sites; Hormone-secreting status associated with a distinct clinical syndrome (functioning NETs); Performance status (PS) 0-1 at presentation, according to the ECOG §	N/A	LM resection (n = 36) (32 were after primary resection)	No resection at all (n = 103) (SSA n = 95, SSA + chemo n = 30, SSA + everolimus n = 14, TACE or RFA + systemic and/or surgical treatment * n = 25)
Du et al. [24]	CN	Retrospective	130	LM from NET.	N/A	Radical resection of primary tumour (n = 42); LM + primary resection (R0) n = 26, LM resection (R0) n = 6; Primary + LM resection n = 26, primary resection n = 42, LM resection n = 6	No resection at all (n = 56) (TACE (16/18 also received an RFA) n = 18, systemic chemotherapy n = 9, SSA n = 12, no treatment n = 17; Chemotherapy (n = 21) chemotherapy (fluorouracil and/or epirubicin and/or doxorubicin and/or etoposide and/or cisplatin, etc.) n = 9, SSA n = 12; TACE (n = 18) (16 also received a RFA)
Bertani et al. [17]	IT	Retrospective	121	Patients with synchronous and unresectable pNET LM.	N/A	Resection of primary tumour (n = 62) (n = 59 also received PRRT)	No resection at all (n = 59) (PRRT n = 55, SSA n = 29)
Boyar et al. [18]	NO	Retrospective	114	Patients with (WHO 2010) grade 1 and grade 2 tumours.	N/A	Resection of primary tumour with curative intent (n = 46)	No resection at all (n = 51) (streptozotocin + 5-fluorouracil/doxorubicin; SSA; IFN; embolization; PRRT; M-tor inhibitor)
Chamberlain et al. [19]	US	Retrospective	85	Patients treated for hepatic NET metastases.	The absence of identifiable liver disease, pathologic review at MSKCC revealing a non-NET or high-grade NET, or a patient decision to seek care elsewhere.	Segmentectomy or enucleation n = 12, lobectomy n = 3, extended resection n = 19 ‡	Chemotherapy (n = 18) (streptozocin + 5-FU; streptozocin + doxorubicin; 5-FU + leucovorin or cisplatin + etoposide); HAE, with polyvinyl alcohol particles (n = 33)
Musunuru et al. [25]	US	Retrospective	48	Patients with liver-only metastatic neuroendocrine tumours.	N/A	Anatomical liver resection n = 6, ablation n = 4, resection and ablation n = 3	Chemotherapy (n = 17) (observation, octreotide, and/or systemic chemotherapy); Embolization (n = 18)

Table 1. *Cont.*

Author	Country	Design	No. Patients (n)	Inclusion Criteria Per Study	Exclusion Criteria Per Study	Intervention Groups	Control Group
Chen et al. [20]	US	Retrospective	38	Patients treated for hepatic NET metastases.	Patients with evidence of extrahepatic disease or unresected known primary tumour.	LM resection (n = 15) (12 were combined with primary resection)	No resection at all (n = 23) (chemoembolization n = 5, chemotherapy and radiation n = 6, chemotherapy only n = 3, radiation only n = 2, no therapy n = 7)
Dousset et al. [23]	FR	Retrospective	34	Patients with metastatic endocrine tumours with bilobar metastases.	N/A	Curative intent resection n = 12 Palliative intent n = 5 †	Chemotherapy (n = 8) (streptozotocin + fluorouracil n = 4, chemoembolization n = 4)
							LTx (n = 9)
Coppa et al. [22]	IT	Retrospective	29	LM from NET, confirmed histological diagnosis.	Non-carcinoid primary tumours, tumours with systemic venous drainage.	Hepatic resection with curative intent (n = 20)	LTx (n = 9)

IFN: interferon, IT: Italy, NO: Norway, US: United States, FR: France, 5-FU: 5-fluoro-uracil, CN: China, DE: Germany, pNET: pancreatic neuroendocrine tumours, NET: neuroendocrine tumours, LM: liver metastases, LTx: liver transplantation, NEN: neuroendocrine neoplasms, N/A: not available, PRRT: peptide receptor radionuclide therapy, RFA: radiofrequency ablation, SSA: somatostatin analogues; TACE: transarterial chemoembolization; * these interventions were also received by patients in the LM resection group; † n = 4 received additional chemotherapy and n = 4 chemoembolization; ‡ 28/34 with a curative intent; § Eastern Cooperative Oncology Group; ¶ Memorial Sloan Kettering Cancer Center.

Table 2. Patient characteristics of included studies.

Study	No. Patients (n)	Sex (n, %) Male	Sex (n, %) Female	Age (Years)	Primary Tumour Location Pancreas (n, %)	Primary Tumour Location Small Bowel (n, %)	Primary Tumour Location Other/Unknown (n, %)	LM Size in cm (Median, Range)	Non-Functional NETs (n, %)	Resection of Primary Tumour (n, %)	Resectable/Unresectable LM	Uni-/Bilobar Metastases	Extrahepatic Disease (n, %)	WHO 2010 Grade
Watzka et al. [27]	204	111 (54)	93 (46)	58 ± 15 (60) *	58 (28)	73 (36)	73 (36)	N/A	123 (61)	165 (81)	Mixed	N/A	N/A	All
Partelli et al. [26]	166	92 (55)	74 (45)	N/A ‡	166	0	0	LM resection 0.8 cm (0.3–1.7 cm); no resection at all 3.4 cm (1–7 cm) †	152 (92)	91 (55)	Resectable	Both	N/A	All
Citterio et al. [21]	139	67 (48)	72 (52)	56 (51–55) †	36 (26)	66 (47)	37 (27)	N/A	0	93 (67)	Mixed	N/A	N/A	1–2
Du et al. [24]	130	69 (53)	61 (47)	49.0 ± 12.1 (N/A) *	85 (65)	7 [5]	38 (30)	Mean 4.1 cm (range 3–15 cm)	100 (77)	68 (52)	Mixed	N/A	N/A	All
Bertani et al. [17]	121	66 (55)	58 (45)	54.6 ± 12.6 (54.5) *	121 (100)	0	0	N/A	29 (24)	63 (52)	Unresectable	N/A	28 (23)	All
Boyar et al. [18]	114	61 (54)	83 (46)	57 (32–83) †	111 (97)	0	3 [3]	N/A	89 (78)	46 (40)	Mixed	N/A	51 (45)	1–2
Chamberlain et al. [19]	85	37 (44)	48 (56)	52 (20–79) †	42 (49)	0	43 (51)	N/A	49 (58)	36 (42)	Mixed	Both	45 (53)	1–2
Musunuru et al. [25]	48	30 (63)	18 (37)	N/A	15 (31)	0	33 (69)	Embolization 8.9 ± 6.1 cm; chemotherapy 3.7 ± 2.9 cm; any resection 4.5 ± 2.3 cm *	N/A	12 (25)	Unclear	Both	0	N/A
Chen et al. [20]	38	24 (63)	14 (37)	N/A ‡	11 (29)	9 (24)	18 (47)	N/A	9 (24)	12 (32)	Mixed	Biobar	0	N/A
Dousset et al. [23]	34	18 (53)	17 (47)	49.5 (29–76) †	17 (50)	9 (26)	8 (24)	N/A	5 (15)	21 (62)	Mixed	Biobar	0	N/A
Coppa 2001 et al. [22]	29	13 (45)	16 (55)	N/A ‡	0	0	29§	N/A	N/A	11 (38)	Mixed	N/A	0	N/A

* mean ± SD (median); † median (range); ‡ Age was reported for each subgroup separately; § 21 have a pancreatic or ileal origin, whilst 8 originated in the lung or rectum; N/A: not available.

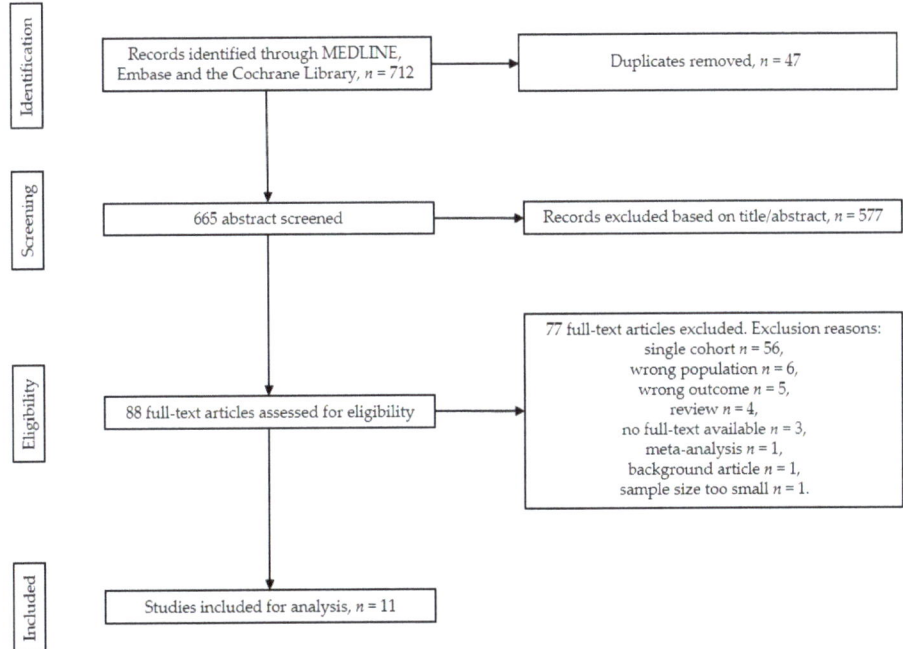

Figure 1. PRISMA flow chart of the study screening and selection process.

3.2. Resection of Primary Tumour versus No Resection at All

This intervention group compares primary resection versus no primary resection with LM presence in both groups. Three studies reported outcomes on resection of primary tumour ($n = 150$) versus no resection of primary tumour ($n = 166$) with a total number of 365 patients [17,18,24]. High statistical heterogeneity based on an I^2 of 92% withheld us from conducting a meta-analysis with these studies (Figure 2).

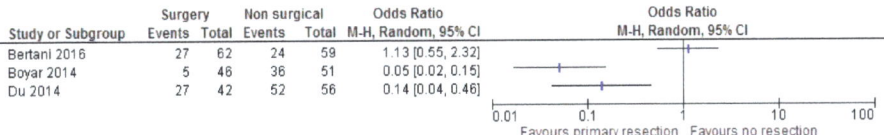

Figure 2. Forest plot for overall survival (OS) after resection of primary tumour versus no resection at all.

3.3. LM Resection versus No Resection at All

Five studies reported outcomes on resection of LM ($n = 139$) versus no resection ($n = 367$) with a total number of 506 patients [20,21,24,26,27]). Chen et al. reported a median DFS of 21 months after LM resection [20]. Partelli et al. reported a median DFS of 42, 27 and 15 months after curative, palliative and no surgery, respectively [26]. Statistical heterogeneity amounted to 75% thus a meta-analysis was performed. The meta-analysis resulted in a statistically significant benefit in 5-year OS (overall survival) in favour of LM resection versus no resection at all (OR 0.15 with 95% CI 0.05–0.42, $p = 0.0003$, Figure 3).

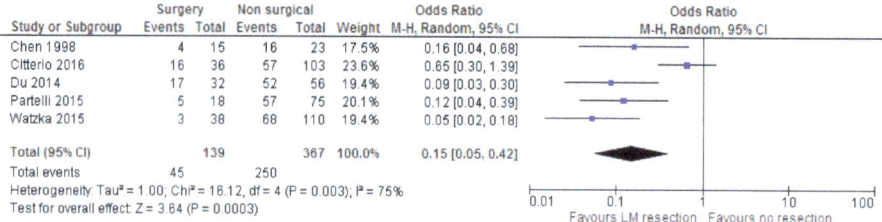

Figure 3. Forest plot for overall survival (OS) after liver metastases (LM) resection versus no resection at all.

3.4. Any Surgery versus Chemotherapy

Four studies reported outcomes on surgery ($n = 138$) versus chemotherapy ($n = 64$) with a total number of 202 patients (19, 23–25). Additional therapy was provided for two out of 32 patients in the surgery group with either TACE or RFA in the study by Du et al. [24]. Statistical heterogeneity amounted to 21%, thus a meta-analysis was performed. The meta-analysis resulted in a statistically significant 5-year OS in favour of any surgery versus chemotherapy (OR 0.05 with 95% CI 0.01–0.21, $p < 0.0001$, Figure 4).

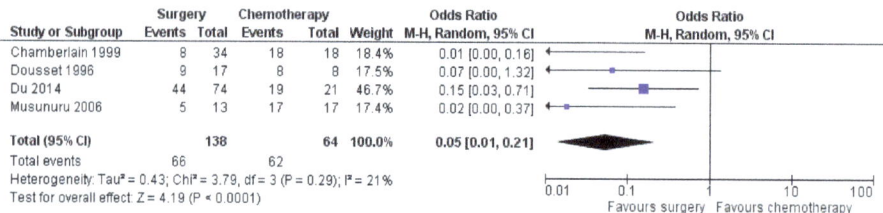

Figure 4. Forest plot for overall survival (OS) after any surgery versus chemotherapy.

3.5. Any Surgery versus Embolization

Three studies reported outcomes on surgery ($n = 121$) versus embolization ($n = 69$) with a total number of 190 patients [19,24,25]. Statistical heterogeneity amounted to 42%, thus a meta-analysis was performed. The meta-analysis resulted in a statistically significant OS in favour of any surgery versus embolization (OR 0.18 with 95% CI 0.05–0.61, $p = 0.006$, Figure 5).

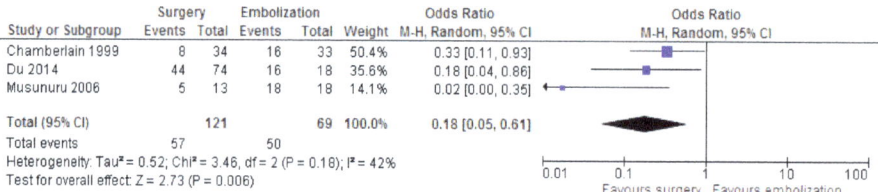

Figure 5. Forest plot for overall survival (OS) after any surgery versus embolization.

3.6. Any Surgery versus LTx

Two studies reported outcomes on surgery ($n = 37$) versus LTx ($n = 18$) with a total number of 55 patients [22,23]. Studies used strict criteria for patients to be eligible for LTx. Statistical heterogeneity amounted to 26%, thus a meta-analysis was performed. The meta-analysis showed no difference in OS regarding any surgery versus LTx (OR 0.69 with 95% CI 0.15–3.14, $p = 0.64$, Figure 6). Coppa et al.

reported a median DFS of 24 months after hepatic resection [22]. Dousset et al. reported a median DFS of 17 months after curative and palliative surgery and 19.5 months after LTx [23].

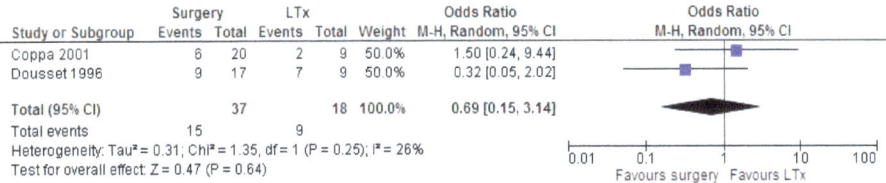

Figure 6. Forest plot for overall survival (OS) after any surgery versus liver transplantation (LTx).

3.7. Risk of Bias

In accordance with the ROBINS-I guidelines, the overall risk of bias was scored as critical for all studies (Table 3), the reason being that all studies scored a critical risk of bias in the 'bias due to confounding' domain due to the lack of randomized controlled trials. The funnel plots show that, as expected, some publication bias is present in the included study (Supplementary Material S2).

Table 3. Risk of bias in included studies scored with the ROBINS-I tool.

	Bias Due to Confounding	Bias in Selection of Participants into the Study	Bias in Classification of Interventions	Bias Due to Deviations from Intended Interventions	Bias Due to Missing Data	Bias in Measurement of Outcomes	Bias in Selection of the Reported Result	Overall Bias
Chamberlain et al. [19]	-	+/-	+	+	+/-	+/-	+/-	-
Coppa et al. [22]	-	+/-	+	+	+/-	+/-	+/-	-
Du et al. [24]	-	+/-	+	+	+/-	+/-	+/-	-
Musunuru et al. [25]	-	+/-	+	+	+/-	+/-	+/-	-
Boyar et al. [18]	-	+/-	+/-	+	+/-	+/-	+/-	-
Bertani et al. [17]	-	+/-	+	+/-	+/-	+/-	+/-	-
Chen et al. [20]	-	+/-	+	+/-	+/-	+/-	+/-	-
Citterio et al. [21]	-	+/-	+	+/-	+/-	+/-	+/-	-
Partelli et al. [26]	-	+/-	+	+/-	+/-	+/-	+/-	-
Watzka et al. [27]	-	+/-	+	+/-	+/-	+/-	+/-	-
Dousset et al. [23]	-	+/-	+/-	+/-	+/-	+/-	+/-	-

+: low (green); +/-: moderate (yellow); -: critical (red).

4. Discussion

Surgical resection of LM with curative intent is the current standard of care [2]. The aim of this treatment strategy is to prolong OS and maintain quality of life. This systematic review presents the first meta-analysis, involving 11 cohort studies and 1108 patients, comparing surgery with other treatment modalities for GEP-NET related LM. The meta-analysis showed a significantly improved 5-year OS after LM resection versus no resection at all, after any surgery versus chemotherapy and after any surgery versus embolization. No significant benefit of any surgery as compared to LTx was observed.

Although our results are heterogeneous, they are supported by a recent study from Yu et al. [28]. In this study, a systematic review and meta-analysis were performed comparing liver resection with non-liver resection treatments for patients with LM from all grades of pNET. The meta-analysis resulted in a median 5-year OS of 68% in the liver resection group, and 27% in the non-liver resection group. Survival outcomes reached statistical significance for 5-year OS with an OR of 5.30 (95% CI [3.24, 8.67] $p < 0.001$), in favour of liver resection.

A number of studies in this systemic review also reported an improved DFS in favour of surgery versus other treatments. However, because of the limited data reported, no meta-analysis could be performed [20,22,23,25]. Data regarding complications was limited, only two studies reported complications due to hepatic surgery [26,27]. Different from an earlier published Cochrane review, cohort studies were considered for inclusion, which enabled the meta-analysis [13]. Although this study was not able to conduct a meta-analysis comparing primary tumour resection to no primary resection, a trend towards a beneficial effect of primary tumour resection is observed and supported by other studies [29,30]. In addition, performing LTx remains a topic of debate due to the small number of patients reported in the literature [31].

This review also included patients with metastases of WHO grade 3 SB-NETs. These patients showed an improved 5-year OS after resection of the LMs. This supports the ENETS 2012 guideline regarding an indication for resection of LM in WHO grade 3 NETs whenever possible, assessed per individual case [2]. We agree with the ENETS 2012 guideline; however, we also propose that the presence of extrahepatic metastases should not be an exclusion criterion, but that resection should be, again, considered per individual case [2]. Our data supports the updated ENETS 2016 guideline, stating that ablative therapies should be considered when surgery is contraindicated in LM from grade 1 and grade 2 NETs (Figure 5) [12].

This systematic review and meta-analysis have a number of limitations, mainly due to the rarity of the disease and limited conducted interventional studies, with a lack of randomized controlled trials (RCT). This resulted in inclusion of 11 retrospective cohort studies, resulting in a low level of evidence (level C) [32]. As a consequence, drawing conclusions is challenging due to a high risk of selection bias, but hypothesis generating remains possible. Moreover, the included studies have small cohort sizes on subgroup level, interventions were performed on different tumour grades and the studies used a variety of types of individual interventional approaches. It is also unfortunate that no quality-of-life data were reported in the included studies. Because our analyses are based only on published data, there is also a risk of publication bias. Despite the obvious drawbacks of this study, it is at present the best available evidence.

Even though a systematic approach was used in this study, the data is of limited quality and the question of which intervention yields the most benefit for OS in patients with LM from pNET/SB-NET remains unanswered. Randomized trials would generate evidence of great quality, but the execution of such a study is challenging (due to the long follow-up time needed and financial burden, among other things). Therefore, further prospective multi-centre research should address this question, for example by collaboration of multiple ENETS Centers of Excellence. Dousset et al. and Partelli et al. also report underestimation of liver disease by preoperative imaging studies, indicating room for improvement [23,26]. Watzka and colleagues reported on the largest included cohort of LM from GEP-NET [27].

In multivariate analysis, occurrence of synchronous or metachronous LM, hormonal activity and the site of the primary tumour were not independent significant prognostic factors, whereas tumour grade and resection margin status were. These prognostics factors should be taken into account when designing new studies.

Currently, a randomized trial is being conducted, comparing the resection of primary tumours vs. no resection of primary tumours in asymptomatic patients with unresectable LM from SB-NET (NCT03442959). However, survival analyses are not expected soon.

Surgical resection of LMs from all grades GEP-NETs should be considered if possible, and chemotherapy and embolization should be considered as an alternative in case surgery is not feasible. We therefore advocate that all patients with LM from pNET/SB-NET should be discussed in referral centers with specialized multidisciplinary meetings for NETs, preferably in ENETS Centers of Excellence.

Supplementary Materials: The following are available online at http://www.mdpi.com/2077-0383/8/3/403/s1, Supplementary Material S1: Search strategy, Supplementary Material S2: Funnel plots.

Author Contributions: Conceptualization: E.K., E.J.M.N.v.D., and A.F.E.; Data curation: E.K.; Formal analysis: E.K. and A.F.E.; Supervision: C.M.H., M.G.H.B., H.-J.K., E.J.M.N.v.D., and A.F.E.; Validation: E.K., C.M.H., H.-J.K., E.J.M.N.v.D., and A.F.E.; Writing—original draft: E.K.; Writing—review and editing: E.K., C.M.H., K.M.A.D., H.-J.K., E.J.M.N.v.D., and A.F.E.

Funding: This research received no external funding.

Acknowledgments: We would like to thank Faridi van Etten-Jamaludin, a clinical librarian, for helping with the electronic searches.

Conflicts of Interest: The authors have no conflict of interest to declare.

References

1. Integraal Kankercentrum Nederland (IKNL). *Cijfers over Kanker*; IKNL: Utrecht, The Netherlands, 2018.
2. Pavel, M.; Baudin, E.; Couvelard, A.; Krenning, E.; Öberg, K.; Steinmüller, T.; Anlauf, M.; Wiedenmann, B.; Salazar, R. ENETS Consensus Guidelines for the Management of Patients with Liver and Other Distant Metastases from Neuroendocrine Neoplasms of Foregut, Midgut, Hindgut, and Unknown Primary. *Neuroendocrinology* **2012**, *95*, 157–176. [CrossRef]
3. Frilling, A.; Sotiropoulos, G.C.; Li, J.; Kornasiewicz, O.; Plöckinger, U. Multimodal management of neuroendocrine liver metastases. *HPB Off. J. Int. Hepato Pancreato Biliary Assoc.* **2010**, *12*, 361–379. [CrossRef]
4. Rinke, A.; Muller, H.H.; Schade-Brittinger, C.; Klose, K.J.; Barth, P.; Wied, M.; Mayer, C.; Aminossadati, B.; Pape, U.F.; Blaker, M.; et al. Placebo-controlled, double-blind, prospective, randomized study on the effect of octreotide LAR in the control of tumor growth in patients with metastatic neuroendocrine midgut tumors: A report from the PROMID Study Group. *J. Clin. Oncol. Off. J. Am. Soc. Clin. Oncol.* **2009**, *27*, 4656–4663. [CrossRef] [PubMed]
5. Caplin, M.E.; Pavel, M.; Ćwikła, J.B.; Phan, A.T.; Raderer, M.; Sedláčková, E.; Cadiot, G.; Wolin, E.M.; Capdevila, J.; Wall, L.; et al. Lanreotide in Metastatic Enteropancreatic Neuroendocrine Tumors. *N. Engl. J. Med.* **2014**, *371*, 224–233. [CrossRef] [PubMed]
6. Ruszniewski, P.; Ish-Shalom, S.; Wymenga, M.; O'Toole, D.; Arnold, R.; Tomassetti, P.; Bax, N.; Caplin, M.; Eriksson, B.; Glaser, B.; et al. Rapid and sustained relief from the symptoms of carcinoid syndrome: Results from an open 6-month study of the 28-day prolonged-release formulation of lanreotide. *Neuroendocrinology* **2004**, *80*, 244–251. [CrossRef]
7. Strosberg, J.; El-Haddad, G.; Wolin, E.; Hendifar, A.; Yao, J.; Chasen, B.; Mittra, E.; Kunz, P.L.; Kulke, M.H.; Jacene, H.; et al. Phase 3 Trial of (177)Lu-Dotatate for Midgut Neuroendocrine Tumors. *N. Engl. J. Med.* **2017**, *376*, 125–135. [CrossRef]
8. Raymond, E.; Dahan, L.; Raoul, J.-L.; Bang, Y.-J.; Borbath, I.; Lombard-Bohas, C.; Valle, J.; Metrakos, P.; Smith, D.; Vinik, A.; et al. Sunitinib Malate for the Treatment of Pancreatic Neuroendocrine Tumors. *N. Engl. J. Med.* **2011**, *364*, 501–513. [CrossRef] [PubMed]
9. Yao, J.C.; Fazio, N.; Singh, S.; Buzzoni, R.; Carnaghi, C.; Wolin, E.; Tomasek, J.; Raderer, M.; Lahner, H.; Voi, M.; et al. Everolimus for the treatment of advanced, non-functional neuroendocrine tumours of the lung or gastrointestinal tract (RADIANT-4): A randomised, placebo-controlled, phase 3 study. *Lancet* **2016**, *387*, 968–977. [CrossRef]
10. Yao, J.C.; Shah, M.H.; Ito, T.; Bohas, C.L.; Wolin, E.M.; Van Cutsem, E.; Hobday, T.J.; Okusaka, T.; Capdevila, J.; de Vries, E.G.; et al. Everolimus for advanced pancreatic neuroendocrine tumors. *N. Engl. J. Med.* **2011**, *364*, 514–523. [CrossRef] [PubMed]
11. Sward, C.; Johanson, V.; Nieveen van Dijkum, E.; Jansson, S.; Nilsson, O.; Wangberg, B.; Ahlman, H.; Kolby, L. Prolonged survival after hepatic artery embolization in patients with midgut carcinoid syndrome. *Br. J. Surg.* **2009**, *96*, 517–521. [CrossRef]
12. Pavel, M.; O'Toole, D.; Costa, F.; Capdevila, J.; Gross, D.; Kianmanesh, R.; Krenning, E.; Knigge, U.; Salazar, R.; Pape, U.F.; et al. ENETS Consensus Guidelines Update for the Management of Distant Metastatic Disease of Intestinal, Pancreatic, Bronchial Neuroendocrine Neoplasms (NEN) and NEN of Unknown Primary Site. *Neuroendocrinology* **2016**, *103*, 172–185. [CrossRef] [PubMed]
13. Gurusamy, K.S.; Ramamoorthy, R.; Sharma, D.; Davidson, B.R. Liver resection versus other treatments for neuroendocrine tumours in patients with resectable liver metastases. *Cochrane Database Syst. Rev.* **2009**, Cd007060. [CrossRef] [PubMed]

14. Ouzzani, M.; Hammady, H.; Fedorowicz, Z.; Elmagarmid, A. Rayyan—A web and mobile app for systematic reviews. *Syst. Rev.* **2016**, *5*, 210. [CrossRef] [PubMed]
15. Figueiredo, M.N.; Maggiori, L.; Gaujoux, S.; Couvelard, A.; Guedj, N.; Ruszniewski, P.; Panis, Y. Surgery for small-bowel neuroendocrine tumors: Is there any benefit of the laparoscopic approach? *Surg. Endosc.* **2014**, *28*, 1720–1726. [CrossRef] [PubMed]
16. Sterne, J.A.C.; Hernán, M.A.; Reeves, B.C.; Savović, J.; Berkman, N.D.; Viswanathan, M.; Henry, D.; Altman, D.G.; Ansari, M.T.; Boutron, I.; et al. ROBINS-I: A tool for assessing risk of bias in non-randomised studies of interventions. *BMJ* **2016**, *355*, i4919. [CrossRef] [PubMed]
17. Bertani, E.; Fazio, N.; Radice, D.; Zardini, C.; Spinoglio, G.; Chiappa, A.; Ribero, D.; Biffi, R.; Partelli, S.; Falconi, M. Assessing the role of primary tumour resection in patients with synchronous unresectable liver metastases from pancreatic neuroendocrine tumour of the body and tail. A propensity score survival evaluation. *Eur. J. Surg. Oncol.* **2017**, *43*, 372–379. [CrossRef] [PubMed]
18. Boyar Cetinkaya, R.; Vatn, M.; Aabakken, L.; Bergestuen, D.S.; Thiis-Evensen, E. Survival and prognostic factors in well-differentiated pancreatic neuroendocrine tumors. *Scand. J. Gastroenterol.* **2014**, *49*, 734–741. [CrossRef] [PubMed]
19. Chamberlain, R.S.; Canes, D.; Brown, K.T.; Saltz, L.; Jarnagin, W.; Fong, Y.; Blumgart, L.H. Hepatic neuroendocrine metastases: Does intervention alter outcomes? *J. Am. Coll. Surg.* **2000**, *190*, 432–445. [CrossRef]
20. Chen, H.; Hardacre, J.M.; Uzar, A.; Cameron, J.L.; Choti, M.A. Isolated liver metastases from neuroendocrine tumors: Does resection prolong survival? *J. Am. Coll. Surg.* **1998**, *187*, 88–92; discussion 92–93. [CrossRef]
21. Citterio, D.; Pusceddu, S.; Facciorusso, A.; Coppa, J.; Milione, M.; Buzzoni, R.; Bongini, M.; deBraud, F.; Mazzaferro, V. Primary tumour resection may improve survival in functional well-differentiated neuroendocrine tumours metastatic to the liver. *Eur. J. Surg. Oncol.* **2017**, *43*, 380–387. [CrossRef] [PubMed]
22. Coppa, J.; Pulvirenti, A.; Schiavo, M.; Romito, R.; Collini, P.; Di Bartolomeo, M.; Fabbri, A.; Regalia, E.; Mazzaferro, V. Resection versus transplantation for liver metastases from neuroendocrine tumors. *Transplant. Proc.* **2001**, *33*, 1537–1539. [CrossRef]
23. Dousset, B.; Saint-Marc, O.; Pitre, J.; Soubrane, O.; Houssin, D.; Chapuis, Y. Metastatic endocrine tumors: Medical treatment, surgical resection, or liver transplantation. *World J. Surg.* **1996**, *20*, 908–914, discussion 914–915. [CrossRef] [PubMed]
24. Du, S.; Wang, Z.; Sang, X.; Lu, X.; Zheng, Y.; Xu, H.; Xu, Y.; Chi, T.; Zhao, H.; Wang, W.; et al. Surgical resection improves the outcome of the patients with neuroendocrine tumor liver metastases: Large data from Asia. *Medicine (Baltimore)* **2015**, *94*, e388. [CrossRef] [PubMed]
25. Musunuru, S.; Chen, H.; Rajpal, S.; Stephani, N.; McDermott, J.C.; Holen, K.; Rikkers, L.F.; Weber, S.M. Metastatic neuroendocrine hepatic tumors: Resection improves survival. *Arch. Surg.* **2006**, *141*, 1000–1004, discussion 1005. [CrossRef]
26. Partelli, S.; Inama, M.; Rinke, A.; Begum, N.; Valente, R.; Fendrich, V.; Tamburrino, D.; Keck, T.; Caplin, M.E.; Bartsch, D.; et al. Long-Term Outcomes of Surgical Management of Pancreatic Neuroendocrine Tumors with Synchronous Liver Metastases. *Neuroendocrinology* **2015**, *102*, 68–76. [CrossRef] [PubMed]
27. Watzka, F.M.; Fottner, C.; Miederer, M.; Schad, A.; Weber, M.M.; Otto, G.; Lang, H.; Musholt, T.J. Surgical therapy of neuroendocrine neoplasm with hepatic metastasis: patient selection and prognosis. *Langenbeck's Arch. Surg.* **2015**, *400*, 349–358. [CrossRef]
28. Yu, X.; Gu, J.; Wu, H.; Fu, D.; Li, J.; Jin, C. Resection of Liver Metastases: A Treatment Provides a Long-Term Survival Benefit for Patients with Advanced Pancreatic Neuroendocrine Tumors: A Systematic Review and Meta-Analysis. *J. Oncol.* **2018**, *2018*, 6273947. [CrossRef]
29. Partelli, S.; Cirocchi, R.; Rancoita, P.M.V.; Muffatti, F.; Andreasi, V.; Crippa, S.; Tamburrino, D.; Falconi, M. A Systematic review and meta-analysis on the role of palliative primary resection for pancreatic neuroendocrine neoplasm with liver metastases. *HPB (Oxford)* **2018**, *20*, 197–203. [CrossRef]
30. Zhou, B.; Zhan, C.; Ding, Y.; Yan, S.; Zheng, S. Role of palliative resection of the primary pancreatic neuroendocrine tumor in patients with unresectable metastatic liver disease: A systematic review and meta-analysis. *OncoTargets Ther.* **2018**, *11*, 975–982. [CrossRef]

31. Moris, D.; Tsilimigras, D.I.; Ntanasis-Stathopoulos, I.; Beal, E.W.; Felekouras, E.; Vernadakis, S.; Fung, J.J.; Pawlik, T.M. Liver transplantation in patients with liver metastases from neuroendocrine tumors: A systematic review. *Surgery* **2017**, *162*, 525–536. [CrossRef] [PubMed]
32. Guyatt, G.H.; Oxman, A.D.; Vist, G.E.; Kunz, R.; Falck-Ytter, Y.; Alonso-Coello, P.; Schünemann, H.J. GRADE: An emerging consensus on rating quality of evidence and strength of recommendations. *BMJ* **2008**, *336*, 924–926. [CrossRef] [PubMed]

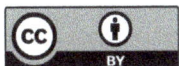

© 2019 by the authors. Licensee MDPI, Basel, Switzerland. This article is an open access article distributed under the terms and conditions of the Creative Commons Attribution (CC BY) license (http://creativecommons.org/licenses/by/4.0/).

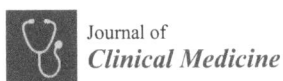

Review

Mixed Neuroendocrine Non-Neuroendocrine Neoplasms: A Systematic Review of a Controversial and Underestimated Diagnosis

Melissa Frizziero [1], Bipasha Chakrabarty [2], Bence Nagy [1], Angela Lamarca [1], Richard A. Hubner [1], Juan W. Valle [1,3] and Mairéad G. McNamara [1,3,*]

1. Department of Medical Oncology, The Christie NHS Foundation Trust, 550 Wilmslow Road, Manchester M20 4BX, UK; Melissa.Frizziero@christie.nhs.uk (M.F.); Bence.Nagy@christie.nhs.uk (B.N.); Angela.Lamarca@christie.nhs.uk (A.L.); Richard.Hubner@christie.nhs.uk (R.A.H.); Juan.Valle@christie.nhs.uk (J.W.V.)
2. Department of Pathology, The Christie NHS Foundation Trust, 550 Wilmslow Road, Manchester M20 4BX, UK; Bipasha.Chakrabarty@christie.nhs.uk
3. Division of Cancer Sciences, University of Manchester, Oxford Road, Manchester M13 9PL, UK
* Correspondence: Mairead.McNamara@christie.nhs.uk

Received: 2 December 2019; Accepted: 16 January 2020; Published: 19 January 2020

Abstract: Mixed neuroendocrine non-neuroendocrine neoplasms (MiNENs) represent a rare diagnosis of the gastro-entero-pancreatic tract. Evidence from the current literature regarding their epidemiology, biology, and management is of variable quality and conflicting. Based on available data, the MiNEN has an aggressive biological behaviour, mostly driven by its (often high-grade) neuroendocrine component, and a dismal prognosis. In most cases, the non-neuroendocrine component is of adenocarcinoma histology. Due to limitations in diagnostic methods and poor awareness within the scientific community, the incidence of MiNENs may be underestimated. In the absence of data from clinical trials, MiNENs are commonly treated according to the standard of care for pure neuroendocrine carcinomas or adenocarcinomas from the same sites of origin, based on the assumption of a biological similarity to their pure counterparts. However, little is known about the molecular aberrations of MiNENs, and their pathogenesis remains controversial; molecular/genetic studies conducted so far point towards a common monoclonal origin of the two components. In addition, mutations in tumour-associated genes, including *TP53*, *BRAF*, and *KRAS*, and microsatellite instability have emerged as potential drivers of MiNENs. This systematic review (91 full manuscripts or abstracts in English language) summarises the current reported literature on clinical, pathological, survival, and molecular/genetic data on MiNENs.

Keywords: mixed non-neuroendocrine neuroendocrine neoplasms; MiNENs; mixed adeno-neuroendocrine carcinoma; MANEC; 2017 WHO classification; 2019 WHO classification

1. Introduction

Epithelial neoplasms displaying a coexistence of a neuroendocrine and non-neuroendocrine histology include a wide spectrum of entities composed of a variable proportion of the two histologies (each representing from 1% to 99% of the tumour mass) and have been described in almost all organs [1,2]. The two components of these mixed neoplasms can exhibit variable morphological features (also depending on the site of origin) as well as degrees of differentiation, and can be combined in different patterns; they can be intimately intermingled within the tumour mass (composite tumours) or they can constitute separate, juxtaposed areas of the tumour mass (collision tumours). In other cases, neuroendocrine and non-neuroendocrine features coexist at a cellular level (amphicrine tumours) [1,3]. Besides their pathological heterogeneity, over the years, mixed neuroendocrine/non-neuroendocrine neoplasms have been assigned a number of different definitions, with some redundant or only partially overlapping (a comprehensive list of the terms used in the literature has been reported by La Rosa et al. [2]), giving rise to a huge inconsistency in published data on these neoplasms.

In 2010, mixed neoplasms from the gastro-entero-pancreatic (GEP) tract containing a neuroendocrine and an exocrine component, each of them present in at least 30% of the tumour mass and being malignant, were classified by the World Health Organisation (WHO) as separate entities and named "mixed adeno-neuroendocrine carcinomas" (MANECs) [4]. The rationale behind the 30% threshold is that a lesser represented component is unlikely to influence the biological behaviour of the whole neoplasm. However, this is an arbitrary threshold and not supported by evidence of its clinical relevance or pathogenic significance [1].

In 2017, the WHO renamed MANECs from the pancreas as "mixed neuroendocrine non-neuroendocrine neoplasms" (MiNENs), where the 30% threshold for each component was maintained, but the term "exocrine" was substituted by the more general term "non-neuroendocrine" to include histological variants that cannot be referred to as exocrine (e.g., squamous or sarcomatoid phenotypes), and the term "carcinoma" was substituted by the term "neoplasm" to recognise the fact that occasionally, one or both components are low-grade malignant [5]. Very recently, the WHO has extended the use of the term to all neoplasms meeting the diagnostic criteria for MiNENs arising from any site within the GEP tract [6]. Compared to "MANECs", the term "MiNENs" is believed to better address the heterogeneous spectrum of possible combinations between neuroendocrine and non-neuroendocrine elements and the variability of morphologies, which are largely determined by the site of origin [2].

Mixed neuroendocrine non-neuroendocrine neoplasms, as per the 2017–2019 WHO definition [5,6], represent an extremely rare diagnosis. According to the Surveillance of Rare Cancers in Europe registry in 2008, the incidence of MiNENs was below 0.01/100,000 cases per annum, and only 96 people were alive with this diagnosis in the whole continent (http://www.rarecare.eu/). Furthermore, evidence from the literature on MiNENs is almost exclusively derived from case reports and small retrospective series. Due to the rarity of this diagnosis, the limited quality of published data, and the use of inconsistent terminology, the epidemiology, prognosis, and best therapeutic management of patients with MiNEN remains unknown.

Based on available evidence, albeit limited and conflicting, the MiNEN is an aggressive entity with a high-grade neuroendocrine component in the majority of cases, and is associated with poor survival outcomes close to those of pure neuroendocrine carcinomas (NECs) [7]. For these reasons, MiNENs are usually treated similarly to their pure NEC counterpart [8]. Alternatively, when the exocrine component is the preponderant and/or most aggressive histology, some clinicians choose to apply the standard of care for adenocarcinomas (ADCs) from the same site of origin [7]. Both practices are based on principles of histological analogy, but are not supported by evidence from prospective randomised trials.

The pathogenesis of MiNENs represents a matter of open debate amongst pathologists and clinicians. Three main theories have been proposed to date [9]: the first theory suggests that the neuroendocrine and non-neuroendocrine components arise independently, in a synchronous or metachronous manner, from distinct precursor cells and merge; the second postulates that the two components derive from a common pluripotent stem cell progenitor, which acquires biphenotypic differentiation during carcinogenesis; a third theory also assumes a common monoclonal origin of the two components, but hypothesises that the neuroendocrine differentiation develops from an initially non-neuroendocrine cell phenotype, through the progressive accumulation of molecular/genetic aberrations, and not vice versa.

The molecular landscape of MiNENs is also poorly understood. A number of studies have recently attempted to identify the key genetic and epigenetic aberrations underlying MiNENs, with a view to better elucidating how this disease develops, and to explore possible biological similarities between its two components, and with their pure counterparts, as well as to identify potential targets for novel therapeutic approaches [10].

This systematic review outlines the epidemiological, clinical, and pathological characteristics and prognosis of GEP-MiNENs, in addition to the most commonly adopted treatment strategies. This review also focuses on reported genetic and epigenetic data, with a view to providing some insights into the biology and pathogenesis of this rare disease.

2. Methods

Biomedical electronic databases, including EMBASE, MEDLINE, and PUBMED, and clinical practice guidelines of the European Neuroendocrine Tumour Society (ENETS), the European Society of Medical Oncology (ESMO), and the National Comprehensive Cancer Network (NCCN) were interrogated for all full manuscripts and conference abstracts written in the English language (at least the abstract), and published between January 2010 (the year of the introduction of the definition of MANEC by WHO [4]) and August 2019, using the following bibliographic search strategy:

"mixed adenoneuroendocrine carcinoma *" or "MANEC *" or "mixed neuroendocrine non-neuroendocrine neoplasm *" or "MiNEN *".

The Preferred Reporting Items for Systematic Reviews and Meta-Analyses (PRISMA) flow diagram for the selection of the studies is reported in Figure 1.

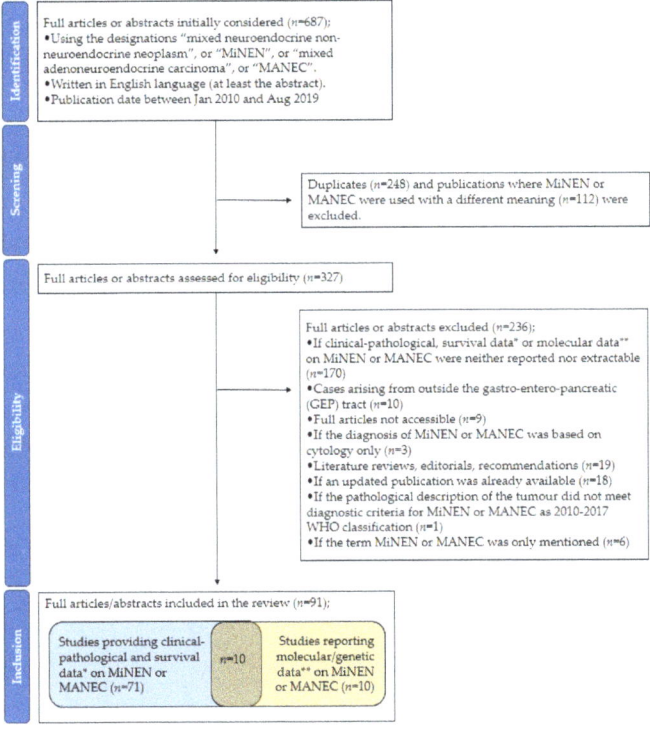

Figure 1. PRISMA flow diagram of study selection. PRISMA = Preferred Reporting Items for Systematic Reviews and Meta-Analyses; n = number of studies; MiNEN = mixed neuroendocrine non-neuroendocrine neoplasm; MANEC = mixed adenoneuroendocrine carcinoma; * follow-up time ≥ 6 months for patients who were alive at the time of publication; ** Immunohistochemical data were not included, except when used to assess DNA mismatch repair protein status.

Studies included were those who met at least one of the following criteria:

- Provision of clinical-pathological and survival data (at least 6 months of follow-up for patients who were alive at the time of publication) on MiNEN or MANEC.
- Molecular/genetic findings on MiNEN or MANEC (immunohistochemical data were not included, except when used for the assessment of DNA Mismatch Repair (MMR) protein status).

Descriptive statistical analyses (e.g., frequencies and medians) were conducted on data extracted from individual studies. Survival data of individual patients presented in case reports (CRs) were pulled and median values (and related 95% confidence intervals) were estimated by applying Kaplan–Meier analysis. In retrospective studies (RSs) where survival data were provided for individual patients (rather than for the whole cohort), estimation of median survival outcomes was attempted by applying Kaplan–Meier analysis. Microsoft Excel and SPSS statistics software were used.

3. Results

A total of 687 publications were screened. Then, 91 (number of patients (n) = 2427 patients) were included [11–101]; 75 publications were full manuscripts, and 16 were conference abstracts. Fifty-five were case reports (CRs) [11–65], and 36 were retrospective studies (RSs) [66–101]. Eighty-four used the term "MANEC" or "mixed adenoneuroendocrine carcinoma", and seven used the term "MiNEN" or "mixed neuroendocrine non-neuroendocrine neoplasm". The number (percentage) of publications per geographical area was as follows; Asia 42 (46.1%), Europe 31 (34.1%), North America 13 (14.3%), South America 2 (2.2%), unknown 3 (3.3%).

3.1. Clinical-Pathological Characteristics, Treatment Modalities, and Survival Outcomes

The site of origin of the primary tumour was as follows; appendix 60.3% (n = 1463), colon–rectum 14.5% (n = 351) (colon 11.2% (n = 272), rectum 1.9% (n = 45), either colon or rectum 1.4% (n = 34)), stomach 6.7% (n = 162), oesophagus/oesophagogastric junction (OGJ) 5.9% (n = 143), pancreas 3.7% (n = 90), biliary tract 1.6% (n = 39), small bowel < 1% (n = 19), anus < 1% (n = 3), unknown primary <1% (n = 3), liver < 1% (n = 1), and GEP non otherwise specified (n.o.s.) 5.9% (n = 144). The remaining nine patients, reported in a study by Apostolidis L. et al. [75], had a MiNEN from outside the GEP tract; data related to these patients could not be selectively extracted and discarded, and therefore were included in the analysis.

Data on gender were provided in 77 studies (n = 983) [11–65,68–70,72–75,79,80,82,84–86,88,93–97,99–101]; 65.6% (n = 645) were male, and 34.4% (n = 338) were female. The frequency of the two genders according to the primary tumour site could be explored in 71 studies (n = 580) [11–65,68,70,72–74,79,80,82,86,88,93–95,97,100,101]. In the majority of subgroups per primary tumour site, the male gender was prevalent; stomach 89.5% (n = 68 out of 976), oesophagus/OGJ 86.1% (n = 87 out of 101), pancreas 66.7% (n = 24 out of 36), colon 63.2% (n = 43 out of 68), rectum 63.1% (n = 12 out of 19), small bowel 60.0% (n = 3 out of 5), anus 100% (n = 2 out of 2), and liver 100% (n = 1 out of 1), whereas among MiNENs from the biliary tract (male 47.8%; n = 11 out of 23) and the appendix (male 51.0%; n = 127 out of 249) the two genders were represented in roughly equal proportions.

The stage of the disease at diagnosis was noted in 77 studies (n = 2117) [11–66,68–70,73–75,79,80,84–88,91,94–96,98–101], and could be classified as follows; localised (Loc), curatively treated, with or without loco-regional nodal involvement, without distant metastases (81.6%; n = 1727); advanced (Adv), not suitable for curative treatment, and with or without distant metastases (18.4%; n = 390).

The quantitative composition of the primary tumour was described in 36 studies (n = 294) [12,15,17,19,21,23–25,27,29,30,34,36,39–41,45,46,48–50,52–54,56,57,59,65,73,74,80,82,84–86,92]; the two components were present in equal proportion in 27.9% (n = 82) of cases, whereas in the remaining 72.1% one of the two histologies was predominant; the neuroendocrine component in 42.2% (n = 124), the non-neuroendocrine component in 29.9% (n = 88).

Among 69 studies ($n = 667$) reporting the grade of differentiation of the neuroendocrine component [11–19,21–29,31–52,54–62,68,71,73–75,79,80,82,84–87,89,91–93,96,97,100,101], a large proportion of MiNENs (92.5%; $n = 617$) had a grade 3 neuroendocrine component, whereas 4.3% ($n = 29$) and 3.1% ($n = 21$) had a grade 1 and a grade 2 neuroendocrine component, respectively. Among MiNENs with a grade 3 neuroendocrine component, the morphological subtype (large cell or small cell) was reported in 25 studies ($n = 241$) [11,19,21,22,28,29,32,35,38,40,41,46,47,49,52,55,57–59,62,79,85,86,89,97], and was large cell in 82.2% ($n = 198$) and small cell in 17.8% ($n = 43$).

The histology of the non-neuroendocrine component was reported in 74 studies ($n = 606$) [11–13,15–62,64,65,68,72–75,79–82,84–87,89,91–93,95–97,101], and was consistent with an adenocarcinoma in 92.2% of cases ($n = 559$) (acinar cell carcinoma in 7.6% ($n = 46$)), an adenoma in 4.5% ($n = 27$), a squamous cell carcinoma in 2.5% ($n = 15$), a hepatocellular carcinoma in < 1% ($n = 1$), and a mixture of an adenocarcinoma and a squamous cell carcinoma in < 1% ($n = 4$). The grade of differentiation of the non-neuroendocrine component was specified in 38 studies ($n = 124$), and was well differentiated in 24.2% ($n = 30$), moderately differentiated in 35.5% ($n = 44$), and poorly differentiated in 39.5% ($n = 49$). In one case, the non-neuroendocrine component was described as occupied by a well-differentiated adenocarcinoma and a moderately differentiated squamous cell carcinoma.

Interestingly, in 43 studies ($n = 61$) where more than one diagnostic sample was available [11,13–28,30,32–34,36–39,41–47,49,50,53,55,59–62,64,65,96], the initial diagnosis from the first sample collected (either cytological or histological) was in keeping with MiNEN or suspicion of MiNEN in 36.1% ($n = 22$) of cases, adenocarcinoma in 36.1% ($n = 22$), poorly differentiated neuroendocrine carcinoma in 21.3% ($n = 13$), and well differentiated neuroendocrine tumour in 6.6% ($n = 4$).

Additional data on clinical-pathological characteristics, treatment modalities, and survival outcomes of patients with a diagnosis of MiNEN are presented in Tables 1–3 and Supplementary Materials Table S1.

Among RSs, 18 ($n = 571$) reported information on treatment modalities [68,69,73–75,78,80,84–86,88,91,94,96,98–101] which is illustrated in Figure 2. The great majority of patients received surgery (92.5%; $n = 528$); 66.9% ($n = 353$) in the curative setting, and 13.8% ($n = 73$) in the palliative setting. For the remaining 19.3% ($n = 102$), the disease stage at the time of the surgery remained unknown.

Among RS, 26 ($n = 2176$) reported on survival outcomes of MiNEN [66,68–70,72–76,78,80,82–88,90,94–96,98–101]; in the localised setting, the median recurrence free survival ranged between 8.6 and 75 months, and the median overall survival ranged between 14 and 75 months; in the advanced setting, the progression free survival was 4.6–5.2 months, and the median overall survival was 10–18 months. In studies where both localised and advanced MiNENs were included or the disease stage was not specified, the median overall survival of the whole population ranged between 10.5 and 78 months.

The histology of synchronous or metachronous distant metastases was reported in 14 studies ($N = 51$) [11,17,22,31,50,57,58,62–64,85,86,92,96], and was consistent with a single or predominant poorly differentiated neuroendocrine component in 60.8% ($n = 31$) of cases, with a mixture of a neuroendocrine carcinoma and an adenocarcinoma in 33.3% ($n = 17$), and a single or predominant adenocarcinoma component in 5.9% ($n = 3$).

Ten studies investigated the prognosis of MiNENs in comparison with other neoplasms from the same sites of origin (Supplementary Table S2); whilst it seems well recognised that patients with an MiNEN diagnosis carry a worse prognosis than patients with well differentiated neuroendocrine tumours [69,70,94,98], it remains controversial whether MiNENs have a better prognosis or not than pure neuroendocrine carcinomas [72,83,85,88,94,96,98,101]. Compared to appendiceal goblet cell carcinoids (more recently defined as goblet cell adenocarcinomas), MiNENs seem to have less favourable survival outcomes [69,70].

Table 1. Clinical-pathological characteristics and survival outcomes of patients with a diagnosis of mixed neuroendocrine non-neuroendocrine neoplasm in case reports.

Characteristics	All Patients (*n* = 61)
Gender	
Male	47 (77.1%)
Female	14 (22.9%)
Age at diagnosis (median)	64 years
Primary tumour site	
Stomach	23 (37.3%)
Oesophagus/OGJ	5 (8.2%)
Pancreas	2 (3.3%)
Biliary tract	15 (24.6%)
Colon	11 (18.0%)
Rectum	3 (4.9%)
Small bowel	1 (1.6%)
Liver	1 (1.6%)
Ki-67 NE component (median)	70% (available for 41 patients)
Disease stage at diagnosis	
Localised	48 (78.7%)
Advanced	13 * (21.3%)
Survival outcomes	
n (%) of patients with survival data	59 (96.7%)
n (%) of recurrence events	18 (37.5%)
n (%) of death events	21 (35.6%)
Follow-up time (median)	14.5 months
Overall Survival (median)	35 months (95%CI could not be estimated)
Sites of recurrence (localised stage cases)	11 †
Liver	7 (63.6%)
Retroperitoneal lymph nodes	2 (18.1%)
Peritoneum	1 (9.0%)
Lung	1 (9.0%)
Supraclavicular lymph node	1 (9.0%)
Scalp	1 (9.0%)
Sites of progression (advanced stage cases)	7 ‡
Liver	5 (71.4%)
Local recurrence after palliative surgery	1 (14.3%)
Not reported	1 (14.3%)

n = number of patients; OGJ = oesophagogastric junction; NE = neuroendocrine; 95%CI = 95% confidence interval; * 31 patients included in survival analysis for the advanced stage subgroup (13 patients with advanced disease at diagnosis plus 18 patients who recurred after initial curative treatment for localised disease); † sites of disease recurrence were reported for 11 out of 18 patients with localised diseases who developed recurrence; ‡ information on disease status at the last follow-up was available for 9 out of 13 patients with advanced disease at diagnosis, and 7 out of these 9 patients had documented progression.

Table 2. Treatment modalities and survival outcomes of patients with a diagnosis of mixed neuroendocrine non-neuroendocrine neoplasm in case reports according to disease stage.

Localised (n = 48)		Advanced (n = 13)	
Primary Tumour Site		**Primary Tumour Site**	
Upper gastro-intestinal tract	25 (52.1%)	Upper gastro-intestinal tract	3 (23.1%)
Lower gastro-intestinal tract	8 (16.7%)	Lower gastro-intestinal tract	7 (53.8%)
Hepato-pancreato-biliary tract	15 (31.2%)	Hepato-pancreato-biliary tract	3 (23.1%)
Curative treatment		**Palliative treatment (n = 31 *)**	
Surgery alone	29 (60.4%)	Surgery alone	2 (6.5%)
Surgery + CT	16 (33.3%)	Surgery + CT	6 (19.4%)
Surgery + CT + RT	3 (6.3%)	CT + RT	2 (6.5%)
		CT alone	9 (29.0%)
		RT alone	2 (6.5%)
		Best supportive care	4 (12.9%)
		Unknown	6 (19.4%)
Curative surgery	48 (100%)	Palliative surgery	8 (25.8%)
Perioperative CT or CT/RT	19 (39.6%)	Palliative CT	17 (54.8%)
CT regimen (+/−RT)		**CT regimen (+/−Surgery +/−RT)**	
Platinum/Etoposide	3 (15.8%)	Platinum/Etoposide	6 (35.3%)
Platinum/Irinotecan	1 (5.2%)	Platinum/Irinotecan	1 (5.9%)
Fluoropyrimidine/Platinum/Irinotecan	1 (5.2%)	Fluoropyrimidine/Platinum	1 (5.9%)
Fluoropyrimidine/Platinum/Etoposide	1 (5.2%)	Fluoropyrimidine/Oxaliplatin (+/−mAb)	3 (17.6%)
Fluoropyrimidine/Oxaliplatin	8 (42.1%)	Fluoropyrimidine/Irinotecan (+/−mAb)	2 (11.8%)
Fluoropyrimidine alone	2 (10.5%)	Fluoropyrimidine alone	1 (5.9%)
Gemcitabine/Oxaliplatin	2 (10.5%)	Gemcitabine	1 (5.9%)
Regimen not specified	1 (5.2%)	Regimen not specified	2 (11.8%)
Non-NE-like regimens	12 (66.7%)	Non-NE-like regimens	8 (53.3%)
NEC-like regimens	4 (22.2%)	NEC-like regimens	7 (46.7%)
Both NEC-like and non-NE-like regimens	2 (11.1%)	Both NEC-like and non-NE-like regimens	0
Median RFS (95%CI) (could be estimated for 48 patients)	36 m (95%CI; 5.8–66.2)	**Median PFS (95%CI)** (could be estimated for 17 patients)	5 m (95%CI; 3.6–6.4)
Median OS (95%CI) (could be estimated for 48 patients)	N.R.	**Median OS (95%CI)** (could be estimated for 20 patients)	12m (95%CI; 4.4–19.6)

n = number of patients; CT = chemotherapy; RT = radiotherapy; Platinum = cisplatin or carboplatin; mAb = monoclonal antibody; NEC-like regimens = regimens recommended for pure neuroendocrine carcinomas; non-NE-like regimens = regimens recommended for pure non-neuroendocrine malignancies (most commonly adenocarcinomas or squamous cell carcinomas) from the same site of origin; RFS = recurrence free survival; PFS = progression free survival; OS = overall survival; m = months; 95%CI = 95% confidence interval. * 13 patients with advanced disease at diagnosis plus 18 patients who relapsed after initial curative treatment.

Table 3. Treatment modalities and survival outcomes of patients with a diagnosis of mixed neuroendocrine non-neuroendocrine neoplasm in retrospective studies.

Reference	Primary Tumour Site	n pts	Age at Diagnosis ‡	n (%) Localised	n (%) Advanced	Ki-67 NE Component ‡	Treatment for Localised Disease	Treatment for Advanced Disease	Median RFS	Median OS (Localised)	Median PFS	Median OS (Advanced)	Median OS (Whole Population)
Shen C., 2016	Stomach	20	62.2 years	14 (70%)	6 (30%)	n.a.	Surgery alone (13; 65%) Surgery + CT (7; 35%) • Platinum/Etop or Platinum-irinotecan	n.a.	n.a.	n.a.	n.a.	n.a.	10.5 m
Lim S.M., 2016	Stomach	17	n.a.	n.a.	n.a.	n.a.	n.a.	n.a.	n.a.	n.a.	n.a.	n.a.	36.4 m
Nie L., 2016	Stomach	14	60.5 years	13 (92.9%)	1 (7.1%)	n.a.	Surgery * (13; 100%)	Surgery * (1; 100%)	N.R. #	N.R. #	not applicable	not applicable	N.R.#
Park J.Y., 2014	Stomach	10	65.5 years	10 (100%)	n.a.	n.a.	Surgery alone (3; 30%) Surgery + CT (7; 70%) • Fluorop alone: 2 • Fluorop/other **: 1 • Fluorop/platinum: 4	n.a.	~75 m @	~75 m @	n.a.	n.a.	~75 m @
Zhang P., 2018	Oesophagus/OGJ	96	62.1 years	82 (85.4%)	14 (14.6%)	66.7%	Surgery * (87; 90.6%)	n.a.	n.a.	n.a.	n.a.	n.a.	73.3 m
van der Veen A., 2018	Stomach (8) Oesophagus/OGJ (9)	17	64.3 years	17 (100%)	n.a.	n.a.	Surgery alone (8; 47%) Surgery + CT (5; 29.4%) • Anthracycline/platinum: 5 Surgery + CT + RT (4; 23.5%) • Platinum/etoposide: 1 • Platinum/taxane: 2 • Other**: 1	n.a.	n.a.	Stomach: ~14 m @ Oesophagus/OGJ: ~44 m @	n.a.	n.a.	Stomach: ~14 m @ Oesophagus/OGJ: ~44 m @
Basturk O., 2014	Pancreas	28	n.a.	n.a.	n.a.	n.a.	n.a.	n.a.	n.a.	n.a.	n.a.	n.a.	44 m
Schimmack S., 2017	Pancreas	11	n.a.	8 (72.7%)	3 (27.3%)	n.a.	n.a.	n.a.	n.a.	n.a.	n.a.	n.a.	60 m
Yang M., 2016	Pancreas	6	47 years	3 (50%)	3 (50%)	n.a.	Surgery * (3; 100%)	Surgery * (3; 100%)	n.a.	n.a.	n.a.	n.a.	15 m
Pop G., 2016	Pancreas	5	n.a.	n.a.	5 (100%)	n.a.	n.a.	Surgery * (5; 100%)	n.a.	n.a.	n.a.	n.a.	10 m
Zheng Z., 2019	Biliary tract	6	62 years	6 (100%)	n.a.	70%	Surgery alone (6; 100%)	n.a.	9.5 m	23 m	n.a.	n.a.	23 m
La Rosa S., 2018	Pancreas	4	n.a.	n.a.	n.a.	n.a.	n.a.	n.a.	n.a.	n.a.	n.a.	n.a.	n.a.
Olevian D., 2015	Colon	26	n.a.	n.a.	n.a.	n.a.	n.a.	n.a.	n.a.	n.a.	n.a.	n.a.	n.a.
Jesinghaus M., 2017	Colon	19	64.3 years	n.a.	n.a.	n.a.	n.a.	n.a.	n.a.	n.a.	n.a.	n.a.	n.a.
Kolasinska-Cwikla AD., 2016	Colon	15	n.a.	n.a.	n.a.	26.9%	Surgery * (15; 100%)		n.a.	n.a.	n.a.	n.a.	26 m
Sinha N., 2018	Colon	14	73.5 years	5 (35.7%)	9 (64.3%)	n.a.	n.a.	n.a.	n.a.	n.a.	n.a.	11 m †	11 m †
Lee S.M., 2016	Colon	8	n.a.	n.a.	5 (100%)	n.a.	n.a.	n.a.	n.a.	n.a.	n.a.	n.a.	n.a.
Bongiovanni M., 2017	Colon	6	n.a.	6 (100%)	n.a.	<2%	Surgery * (6; 100%)	n.a.	n.a.	n.a.	n.a.	n.a.	n.a.
Woischke C., 2017	Colon (10) Rectum (5)	15	72 years	n.a.	n.a.	71%	Surgery alone (1; 25%) Surgery + CT (3; 75%) • Fluorop alone: 3	n.a.	n.a.	n.a.	n.a.	n.a.	n.a.
Komatsubara T., 2016	Colon (5) Rectum (1)	6	69 years	4 (66.7%)	2 (33.3%)	50%	Surgery + CT (2; 100%) • Fluorop alone: 1 • Fluorop/Irinotecan: 1	n.a.	n.a.	n.a.	n.a.	n.a.	53 m *

Table 3. Cont.

Reference	Primary Tumour Site	n pts	Age at Diagnosis ‡	n (%) Localised	n (%) Advanced	Ki-67 NE Component ‡	Treatment for Localised Disease	Treatment for Advanced Disease	Median RFS	Median OS (Localised)	Median PFS	Median OS (Advanced)	Median OS (Whole Population)
Brathwaite S., 2016	Appendix	249	58 years	176 (70.7%)	73 (29.3%)	n.a.	n.a.	n.a.	n.a.	n.a.	n.a.	18 m	78 m
Mehrvarz Sarshekeh A., 2016	Appendix	1173	n.a.	1034 (88.2%)	139 (11.8%)	n.a.	n.a.	n.a.	n.a.	Stage I (52 m), Stage II (43 m), Stage III (28 m)	n.a.	17 m	17 m (stage IV)–52 m (stage I)
Milione M., 2018	Stomach (32) Oesophagus/OGJ (12) Pancreas (14) Biliary tract (10) Colon (74) Rectum (18)	160	n.a.	143 (89.4%)	17 (10.6%)	≥55%: 82.5% <55%: 17.5%	Surgery * (143; 100%)	Surgery * (17; 100%)	n.a.	n.a.	n.a.	n.a.	13.2 m
Yin X.N., 2018	Stomach (20) Rectum (6) Small bowel (4) Appendix (1)	31	61 years	27	4	n.a.	Surgery * (27; 100%)	Surgery * (4; 100%)	n.a.	n.a.	n.a.	n.a.	13 m @
Apostolidis L., 2018	Stomach (6) Oesophagus/OGJ (11) Pancreas (14) Biliary tract (4) Colon-rectum (44) Small bowel (6) Anus (1) Non-GEP (9)	96	59 years	61 (63.5%)	35 (36.5%) (68 for survival analysis)	78%	Surgery alone (23; 37.7%) Surgery + CT ** (25; 40.9%) Surgery + CT + RT ** (9; 14.8%) Unknown treatment (4; 6.6%)	CT alone (54; 79.4%) • NEC-like: 31 • ADC-like: 23 Unknown treatment (14; 20.6%)	8.6 m (surgery alone) – 12.9 m (surgery + periop)	18.9 m (surgery alone) – 75m (surgery + periop)	5.2 m	17.4 m	44.5 m
Düzköylü Y., 2018	Stomach (5) Pancreas (1) Biliary tract (2) Colon (1) Rectum (1)	10	67.5 years	9 (90%)	1 (10%)	55.5%	Surgery * (5; 55.67%) Surgery + CT ** (4; 44.4%)	Surgery + CT ** (1; 100%)	n.a.	N.R.#	n.a.	n.a.	N.R.#
Frizziero M., 2017	Stomach (3) Oesophagus/OGJ (10) Pancreas (3) Biliary tract (2) Colon-rectum (31) Small bowel (3) Unknown (1)	53	62 years	28 (52.8%)	25 (47.2%) (41 for survival analysis)	70%	Surgery alone (12; 42.9%) Surgery + CT ** (7; 25%) Surgery + CT + RT ** (7; 25%) CT + KT (1; 3.6%) Unknown treatment (1; 3.6%)	CT alone (27; 65.9%) • Platinum-based: 20 • Irinotecan-based: 3 • Gemcitabine: 1 • Others **: 3 CT + RT (1; 2.4%) RT alone (1; 2.4%) Best Supportive care (11; 26.8%) Unknown treatment (1; 2.4%)	19.4 m	21 m	4.6 m	13.6 m	18.6 m
La Rosa S., 2018	Stomach (2) Colon (4) Rectum (5) Small bowel (3)	14	57.5 years	n.a.	n.a.	1%	n.a.	n.a.	n.a.	n.a.	n.a.	n.a.	N.R.#
Scardoni M., 2014	Stomach (2) Pancreas (2) Rectum (1) Small bowel (1)	6	68 years	n.a.	n.a.	65%	n.a.	n.a.	n.a.	n.a.	n.a.	n.a.	n.a.
Dulskas A., 2019	Colon (4) Rectum (3) Anus (2)	9	61 years	3 (33.3%)	6 (66.7%)	65%	Surgery alone (2; 66.7%) Surgery + CT + KT (1; 33.3%)	• Fluorop/Oxaliplatin: 3 • Platinum/Etoposide: 2 • Fluorop alone: 1 Surgery alone (1; 16.7%) Surgery + CT (3; 6%) Surgery + CT + KT (1; 20%) CT + KT (1; 60%)	n.a.	n.a.	n.a.	n.a.	N.R.#
Spada F., 2019	Colon-rectum (32) GEP n.o.s. (19)	51	n.a.	n.a.	n.a.	n.a.	n.a.	n.a.	n.a.	n.a.	n.a.	n.a.	14.4 m

Table 3. Cont.

Reference	Primary Tumour Site	n pts	Age at Diagnosis ‡	n (%) Localised	n (%) Advanced	Ki-67 NE Component ‡	Treatment for Localised Disease	Treatment for Advanced Disease	Median RFS	Median OS (Localised)	Median PFS	Median OS (Advanced)	Median OS (Whole Population)
Brathwaite S., 2016	Colon (4) Appendix (40) Small bowel (1) Unknown (1)	46	54 years	15 (32.6%)	31 (67.4%)	n.a.	Surgery alone (7; 46.7%) Surgery + CT ** (8; 53.3%)	Surgery alone (6; 19.4%) Surgery + CT ** (23; 74.2%) Unknown treatment (2; 6.4%)	n.a.	n.a.	n.a.	n.a.	49.2 m
Bu S., 2017	GEP n.o.s.	19	n.a.	n.a.	n.a.	n.a.	n.a.	n.a.	n.a.	n.a.	n.a.	n.a.	25 m @
Melchior L.C., 2019	GEP n.o.s.	43	n.a.	n.a.	n.a.	n.a.	n.a.	n.a.	n.a.	n.a.	n.a.	n.a.	n.a.
Sahnane N., 2015	GEP n.o.s.	36	n.a.	n.a.	n.a.	n.a.	n.a.	n.a.	n.a.	n.a.	n.a.	n.a.	n.a.
Yang H.-M., 2015	GEP n.o.s.	27	n.a.	n.a.	n.a.	n.a.	n.a.	n.a.	n.a.	n.a.	n.a.	n.a.	n.a.

n = number; Fluorop = fluoropyrimidine; CT = chemotherapy; RT = radiotherapy; periop = perioperative CT and/or RT; OGJ = oesophagogastric junction; GEP = gastroenteropancreatic tract; n.o.s. = not otherwise specified (primary tumour arising within the gastroenteropancreatic tract but the exact organ of origin was not specified or could not be extracted); NE = neuroendocrine; NEC = neuroendocrine carcinoma; ADC = adenocarcinoma; n.a. = information not available or could not be extracted; N.R.# = not reached (further information provided in supplementary Table S1); RFS = recurrence free survival; PFS = progression free survival; OS = overall survival; m = months; ‡ mean or median; * unknown whether any perioperative treatment; ** regimen not specified; † survival estimated by applying Kaplan-Meier analysis to data provided in the publication; @ survival estimation extracted from Kaplan–Meier curves.

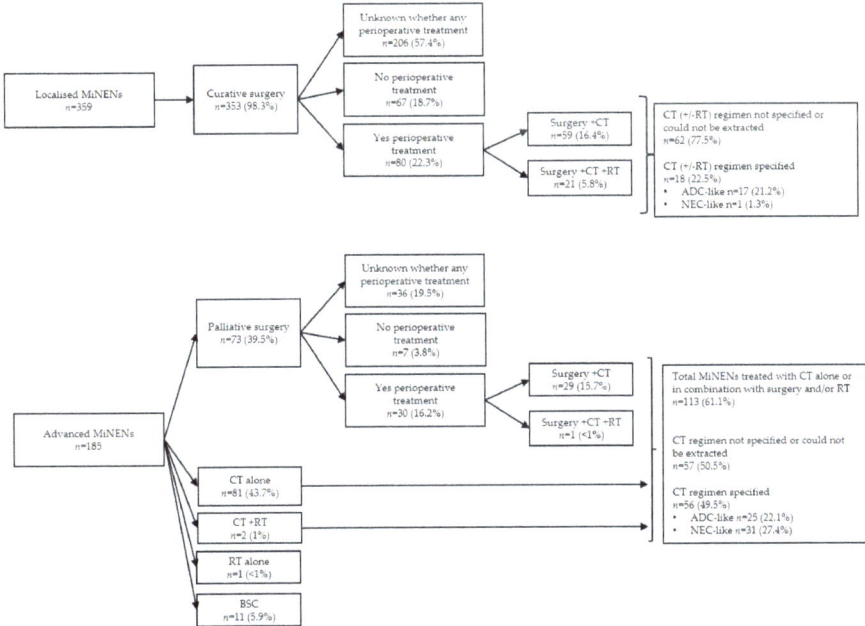

Figure 2. Treatment modalities of MiNEN in retrospective studies. MiNEN = mixed neuroendocrine non-neuroendocrine neoplasm; *n* = number of patients; CT = chemotherapy; RT = radiotherapy; BSC = best supportive care; peri operative = pre surgical and/or post-surgical; ADC-like = in keeping with standard of care for pure adenocarcinomas from the same sites of origin; NEC-like = in keeping with standard of care for pure neuroendocrine carcinomas.

3.2. The Molecular Landscape of MiNEN and Pathogenetic Hypotheses

Twenty studies (*n* = 381) reported on the genetic/molecular alterations underlying MiNEN [29,30,35,58,59,64,67,71,72,77,79,81,82,85,89,91–93,95,97]. In 49.1% of cases where genetic/molecular data was available, the site of origin of MiNEN was the colon–rectum. Most frequent alterations in MiNEN involved well-characterised cancer gene drivers and/or their protein products, such as *TP53* (tumour protein p53), *RB1* (retinoblastoma tumour corepressor 1), *PTEN* (phosphatase and tensin homolog), *APC* (adenomatous polyposis coli), *PI3KCA* (phosphatidylinositol-4,5-bisphosphate 3-kinase catalytic subunit alpha), *KRAS* (Kirsten rat sarcoma viral oncogene homolog), *BRAF* (v-raf murine sarcoma viral oncogene homolog B), and MYC (v-myc avian myelocytomatosis viral oncogene homolog) [frequencies of these alterations in individual studies are presented in Table 4]. Activation of the prostaglandin E2 receptor 4 (PTGER4) [95], and microsatellite instability (MSI) have also been proposed as putative driver events of MiNEN.

Table 4. Molecular data on patients with mixed neuroendocrine non-neuroendocrine neoplasms.

Reference	Primary Tumour Site	n pts	Method(s)	Molecular Findings
Fujita Y., 2019	Stomach	1	PCR, DNA methylation analysis	*TP53* mutation: absent in either components. Low DNA methylation status in either components. Allele imbalance (AI) on chromosomes 5q, 8p, 11q and 22q in NEC, AI on chromosome 11q in ADC.
Farooq F., 2018	Stomach	1	Targeted NGS (255 cancer-related genes—Foundation Medicine)	Tumour with trilineage differentiation (NEC, ADC, SCC) *KRAS, NF1, CDKN2A/B, TP53* mutations: present in all 3 components (same mutation). MSI status: negative in all 3 components. Low TMB in all 3 components. *CDK6, PIK3CG, TOP2A* amplification: present only in NEC. Loss of *PTEN* exons 1–2: present in ADC and SCC (not in NEC). *NOTCH1* mutation: present only in ADC *TERT* amplification: present only in SCC.
Yuan W., 2017	Oesophagus/OGJ	2	Whole exome sequencing, whole genome single nucleotide polymorphism	Multiregional next-generation sequencing *TP53* and *NOTCH1* mutation: present in 2/2 (100%)—all regions analysed. *RB1* deletion or LOH: present in 2/2 (100%)—all regions analysed. *PI3KCA, PTEN, KRAS, SOX2, DVL3, TP63* amplification: present in 2/2 (100%)—all regions analysed.
Basturk O., 2014	Pancreas	6	Not specified	*KRAS* mutation: present in 0/6 (0%).
La Rosa S., 2018	Pancreas	4	Fluorescent in situ hybridisation (FISH)	*MYC* amplification and/or chromosome 8 polysomy: present in all 4 cases.
Vanacker L., 2014	Colon	1	Whole exome sequencing, IHC for MMR proteins	*KRAS, APC, BCL9, FOXP1* mutations: present in both components. *SMARC4A* mutation: present only in NEC. MSI status: negative.
Ito H., 2014	Colon	1	Not specified	*KRAS* mutation: absent (analysed in ADC).
Olevian D., 2015	Colon	26	Not specified	*KRAS* mutation: present in 4 (15.4%). *BRAF* mutation: present in 17 (65.4%).
Jesinghaus M., 2017	Colon	19	Targeted NGS (panel including 196 amplicons covering 32 genes)	*TP53* mutation: present in 9 (47.4%). *KRAS* mutation: present in 4 (21.0%). *BRAF* mutation: present in 7 (36.8%). *APC* mutation: present in 3 (15.8%).*RB1* mutation: present in 1 (5.3%). *PTEN* mutation: present in 2 (10.5%). *ATM* mutation: present in 3 (15.8%). *FBXW7* mutation: present in 3 (15.8%). *SOX9* mutation: present in 2 (10.5%). *MYC* amplification: present in 1 (5.3%). MSI status: positive in 2 (10.5%).
Sinha N., 2018	Colon	14	Genome-wide copy number aberration analysis and FISH	*BRAF* mutation: present in 8 (57.1%). *PTGER4* amplification: present in 1 (7.1%). *MYC* amplification: present in 1 (7.1%). MSI status: positive in 1 (7.1%). CN gains of chr.: 5p; 10/14 (71.4%), 7; 11/14 (78.6%), 8q; 12/14 (85.7%), 13q; 9/14 (64.3%), 20q; 11/14 (78.6%). CN losses of chr.: 3p; 5/14 (35.7%), 4p; 7/14 (50%), 8p; 6/14 (42.9%), 18q; 7/14 (50%).

Table 4. Cont.

Reference	Primary Tumour Site	n pts	Method(s)	Molecular Findings
Lee S.M., 2016	Colon	8	Targeted NGS panel analysing substitutions and small indels in 46/50/409 cancer-related genes	TP53 mutation: present in 3 (37.5%). KRAS mutation: present in 6 (75%). BRAF mutation: present in 1 (12.5%). APC mutation: present in 3 (37.5%). RB1 mutation: present in 1 (12.5%). PTEN mutation: present in 1 (12.5%). PI3KCA mutation: present in 1 (12.5%). GNAS mutation: present in 1 (12.5%). SMO mutation: present in 1 (12.5%). FBXW7, CDKN2A, ERBB2, FGFR3, PTPN11 mutation: present in 0 (0%).
Bongiovanni M., 2017	Colon	6	Direct sequencing (not specified)	KRAS, BRAF, PI3KCA mutation: present in 0/6 (0%)—absent in either component. MSI status: positive in 0/6 (0%)—absent in either component.
Woischke C., 2017	Colon (10) Rectum (5)	15	PCR, targeted NGS (50 gene panel) and whole exome sequencing	KRAS mutation assessed by PCR (in 15 patients): present in 9 (60%). Genes assessed by an NGS panel (in 10 patients): TP53 mutation: present in 10 (100%) (same mutation in both components: 6/10, distinct mutations in the two components: 2/10, exclusively in NEC: 1/10, exclusively in ADC: in 1/10). KRAS mutation: present in 9 (90%) (same mutation in both components: 8/9, exclusively in NEC: 1/9). BRAF mutation: present in 2 (20%) (same mutation in both components: 1/2, distinct mutations in the two components: 1/2). APC mutation: present in 8 (80%) (same mutation in both components: 7/8, exclusively in NEC: 1/8). RB1 mutation: present in 3 (30%) (same mutation in both components: 1/3, distinct mutations in the two components: 1/3, exclusively in NEC: 1/3). PI3KCA mutation: present in 5 (50%) (exclusively in ADC: 4/5, exclusively in NEC: 1/5). MET mutation: present in 4 (40%) (same mutation in both components: 1/4, exclusively in NEC: 2/4, exclusively in ADC: 1/4). NOTCH1 mutation: present in 3 (30%) (same mutation in both components: 1/3, exclusively in NEC: 2/3). RET mutation: present in 2 (20%) (same mutation in both components: 1/2, exclusively present in NEC: 1/2).
Quaas A., 2018	Small Bowel	1	Targeted panel including 14 genes and 14 microsatellite loci	Germline BRCA-1 mutation: present. MSI status: absent. TP53 mutation: present. KRAS, NRAS, HRAS, BRAF, DDR2, ERBB2, KEAP1, NFE2L2, PIK3CA, PTEN, RHO, BRCA2 mutations: absent.

Table 4. Cont.

Reference	Primary Tumour Site	n pts	Method(s)	Molecular Findings
Milione M., 2018	Stomach (32)Oesophagus/OGJ (12)Pancreas (14)Biliary tract (10)Colon (74)Rectum (18)	160	PCR, targeted NGS panel	*TP53* mutation (assessed in 71 patients): present in 17 (23.9%) (assessed in the whole tumour). *KRAS* mutation (assessed in 71 patients): present in 12 (16.9%) (assessed in the whole tumour). *BRAF* mutation (assessed in 71 patients): present in 4 (5.6%) (assessed in the whole tumour). MSI status (assessed in 160 patients): positive in 8 (5%) (in both components).
La Rosa S., 2018	Colon (1)Rectum (3)	4	Direct sequencing (not specified)	*KRAS* mutation: present in 0% (in both components). *TP53* mutation: present in 0% (in both components). *PI3KCA* mutation: present in 0% (in both components). MSI status: positive in 0% (in both components).
Scardoni M., 2014	Stomach (2)Pancreas (2)Rectum (1)Small bowel (1)	6	Targeted NGS (54 gene panel)	*TP53* mutation: present in 6 (100%) (5/6 in both components, same mutation; 1/6 only in ADC). *KRAS* mutation: present in 1 (16.7%) (in both components, same mutation). *RB1* mutation: present in 1 (16.7%) (in both components, same mutation). *ERBB4, ATM, JAK3, KDR* mutations: present in 1/6 (16.7%) (only in NEC). *CTNNB1* mutation: present in 1/6 (16.7%) only in ADC. *ATRX, DAXX, MEN1, TSC2* mutations: present in 0/6 (0%).
Melchior L.C., 2019	GEP n.o.s	43	Targeted NGS (50 gene panel)	*TP53* mutation: present in 28 (65.1%). *KRAS* mutation: present in 7 (16.3%). *BRAF* mutation: present in 6 (13.9%).
Sahnane N., 2015	GEP n.o.s	36	PCR, DNA methylation analysis of 34 gene promoters and MMR genes	*KRAS* mutation (assessed in 88 MiNEN and NEC): present in 15 (17%). *BRAF* mutation (assessed in 88 MiNEN and NEC): present in 6 (6.8%) (6 colorectal). Methylation status (assessed in 89 MiNEN and NEC): high levels (>8 methylated genes) in 28 (31.5%). MSI status (assessed in 36 MINEN): positive in 4 (11.1%) (2 stomach and 2 colorectal).
Yang H.-M., 2015	GEP n.o.s	27	Direct sequencing (not specified)	*TP53* mutation: present in 19 (70.4%) (shared by both components in 13/19, only present in NEC in 6/19). *KRAS* mutation: present in 10 (37%) (in both components).

n = number; pts = patients; NEC = neuroendocrine carcinoma; ADC = adenocarcinoma; SCC = squamous cell carcinoma; GEP = gastro-enteropancreatic tract; n.o.s. = non-otherwise specified; OGJ = oesophagogastric junction; MSI = microsatellite instability; MMR = mismatch repair; NGS = next-generation sequencing; PCR = polymerase chain reaction; IHC = immunohistochemistry; CN = copy number; chr. = chromosome. MSI status is defined as positive if MSI is detected by PCR in at least two of the microsatellite loci analysed, or if at least one of the MMR proteins (Mlh1, Msh2, Msh6 or Pms2) is not expressed or abnormally expressed on IHC.

In the majority of cases where the neuroendocrine and non-neuroendocrine components of MiNEN could be analysed separately, the two components exhibited a core of common alterations, supporting the hypothesis of their common clonal origin, but also alterations exclusively present in one or the other the two components [29,30,58,79,95,97], suggesting that at some point of the tumourigenic process, two distinct morphology entities emerge through the activation of separate genetic programmes. Usually, shared mutations involved well-characterised cancer drivers (e.g., *TP53*, *APC*, *KRAS*, *BRAF*) and have higher allele frequencies (compared to alterations which are exclusive of a single component), suggesting their occurrence in the earlier stages of the development of MiNENs [29,58,79,93,97]. In support of this, Yuan et al. performed multiregional next-generation sequencing analysis on samples from spatially separated regions from two patients with oesophageal MiNEN to interrogate intra-tumour heterogeneity and clonal evolution; alterations in *TP53, RB1, PTEN, PI3KCA,* and *KRAS* were identified in all tumour samples/regions from both patients and had higher allele frequencies (compared to alterations not present in all samples/regions). The authors defined these alterations as 'trunk', as they were shared by all tumour clones and were likely involved in initiating the tumourigenic process [35]. Compared to the non-neuroendocrine component, the neuroendocrine component usually carried a higher number of aberrations and a higher allele imbalance [30,58,97], which are suggestive of a more aggressive biology. Some authors postulated that the non-neuroendocrine component may give rise to the neuroendocrine component through a trans-differentiation process and the acquisition of a more aggressive phenotype [30,58,81]. c-Myc and SMARC4A have been indicated as potential mediators of this trans-differentiation process [58,81]. In some cases, the two components exhibited fairly distinct patterns of genetic or chromosomal alterations [93,95,97], raising the possibility of a polyclonal origin for at least a subtype of MiNENs. Interestingly, in the study by La Rosa et al. including only MiNENs composed of an adenoma and a well-differentiated neuroendocrine component, no *KRAS, BRAF,* or *PI3KCA* mutation or MSI was found in either components of all four samples analysed [82].

With regards to the comparison between MiNENs and their pure counterparts at a genetic/molecular level, Sinha et al. reported that colonic MiNENs ($n = 14$) and pure colonic adenocarcinomas ($n = 269$) shared a largely similar copy number aberration (CNA) profile, whereas pure colonic neuroendocrine carcinomas ($n = 5$) displayed distinct structural chromosomal alterations, suggesting that MiNENs may have a closer developmental relationship to adenocarcinomas than to neuroendocrine carcinomas [95]. Likewise, Jesinghaus et al. reported that colorectal MiNENs ($n = 19$) exhibited a genetic/molecular profile broadly similar to that of pure colorectal adenocarcinomas, but lack alterations commonly related to pure neuroendocrine carcinomas of various origins [79].

4. Discussion

This systematic review comprises the largest collection of studies on MiNEN available in the current literature. Overall, evidence available is of poor quality; the studies included are CRs or RSs (neither published nor ongoing (https://clinicaltrials.gov/) prospective trials specifically recruiting patients with a diagnosis of MiNEN were identified), and are extremely heterogeneous in terms of site of origin of the primary tumour, disease stage, geographical area of patients included, and type of information provided (clinical-pathological data, treatment modalities, survival outcomes, genomic/molecular findings). Furthermore, the 2010 WHO classification was ambiguous as to whether adenocarcinomas ex-goblet cell carcinoids (goblet cell carcinoids Tang B and C) could be regarded, or not, as MANEC [4], generating an additional source of inconsistency within the published literature. Therefore, it was not possible to completely rule out the inclusion of these entities in the RSs of the present review, especially in the two largest reporting on appendiceal MiNEN by Brathwaite et al. ($n = 249$) and by Mehrvarz Sarshekeh et al. ($n = 1173$), and this may have introduced a further confounding element.

Acknowledging these limitations, this review suggests that the biological behaviour of MiNENs is mostly driven by the neuroendocrine component, which is poorly differentiated in approximately 90% of cases, and often occupies the distant metastatic sites. This was also corroborated by molecular findings showing that the neuroendocrine component exhibits more genetic and chromosomal alterations.

Regarding treatment modalities, surgery was the treatment of choice for nearly all potentially curable cases, and was also offered to approximately a quarter to a third of patients with advanced disease. In the latter setting, surgery was pursued for symptom relief or with initial curative intent in patients subsequently found to have advanced disease. However, in most cases, the reasons supporting the choice for surgery in the palliative setting remains unknown. Adjuvant, neoadjuvant, or perioperative therapies were offered to a third of patients receiving curative surgery. The choice of perioperative chemotherapy regimen was most often based on the clinical practice guidelines for early stage adenocarcinomas from the same sites of origin; in fact, the use of (neo) adjuvant chemotherapy protocols to prevent/delay the relapse of the neuroendocrine component is not supported by randomised evidence from the perioperative setting of pure grade 2 or 3 neuroendocrine neoplasms [8]. Palliative chemotherapy was delivered to between a half and two thirds of patients with advanced disease, as upfront treatment, or after palliative surgery. Regimens of palliative systemic treatments were chosen according to the standard of care for either pure adenocarcinomas or neuroendocrine carcinomas from the same site of origin in roughly equal proportion. Noticeably, among the clinical practice guidelines from international oncology societies screened, only the ENETS guidelines provide indications on the treatment for patients with a MiNEN diagnosis, and suggest treatment algorithms based on those used in pure neuroendocrine carcinomas [8], probably because of the aggressiveness of the neuroendocrine component in the majority of cases.

Survival outcomes in the localised setting were largely variable across RSs, ranging from a few months to several years, likely due to differences in patient selection criteria and follow-up time. Often, median survival times were not reached in the localised setting due to the lack of long-term follow-up data. This is also reflected in the initial paper selection of the review, where a large proportion of publications was discarded because information on the patient/disease status was completely missing or limited to a short period (<6 months) after initial diagnosis; longer follow-up data should be obtained when reporting on patients with MiNENs to allow for a more reliable estimation of the prognosis of this disease, especially when still potentially curable. In contrast, in the advanced setting, survival outcomes were more consistent across RSs and with those estimated for CRs (median progression free survival of 5–6 months and a median overall survival of 12–18 months), and very close to those of advanced pure neuroendocrine carcinomas [8]. This further supports the putative similarity in biological behaviour between MiNENs and pure neuroendocrine carcinomas in the advanced setting.

The limitation of biopsy samples in diagnosing MiNENs is a critical issue. Biopsies may not accurately distinguish MiNENs from their pure counterparts, especially because this discrimination depends on a quantitative threshold. In fact, in the present review, the initial biopsy was able to identify the presence of a mixed histology in only a third of cases. This can be due to either the paucity of tumour tissue in the biopsy sample, not representative of both histologies, or because the biopsy is performed on metastatic site, most commonly occupied by only one of the two components. As a further demonstration, in the current review, only around 1 out of 5 patients presented with advanced stage at diagnosis; a much higher proportion of advanced cases would be expected for a highly aggressive disease, and this may be due to the limited ability of biopsy to diagnose advanced MiNENs when not amenable to surgical resection. There is also controversy surrounding the validity of the 30% threshold as discriminatory criterion between MANECs/MiNENs and their pure counterparts. Whether the presence of elements with neuroendocrine differentiation within predominantly exocrine neoplasms, or vice versa, affects the outcome of patients and informs clinical decision making, and whether specific cut-offs in the proportions of each component account for different prognoses and responses to treatment, represent unanswered questions. Some studies have demonstrated that alternative thresholds (e.g., < versus > 10% or 20%) identify adenocarcinomas associated with a minor neuroendocrine component as having a significantly better prognosis than neoplasms with a proportion of neuroendocrine component above those thresholds [86,88]. La Rosa et al. proposed a solution to partially overcome this issue [2]; they suggested that if there is a suspicion of a mixed neuroendocrine/non-neuroendocrine neoplasm within a tumour sample, further confirmation should be pursued through immunohistochemical analysis.

Studies reporting on molecular/genetic data of GEP MiNENs have identified well-characterised carcinogenetic hallmarks of more common GEP malignancies as potential drivers of this disease, such as alterations affecting *TP53, KRAS, BRAF, APC, PI3KCA*, and MSI [102], corroborating what was previously reported by Girardi D.M. et al. [10]; these alterations are usually shared between the two components and likely present in founding clones. Although displaying a biological behaviour more similar to that of pure neuroendocrine carcinomas, the molecular/genetic landscape of GEP MiNENs seems to be closer to that of pure adenocarcinomas. This supports the hypothesis according to which the two components of MiNEN may arise from common glandular precursor through similar sequences of aberrant events to those driving pure GEP adenocarcinomas [79,97]. At a later stage of the tumorigenesis, the two components separate and evolve independently, with the neuroendocrine one accumulating more aberrations and acquiring a more lethal phenotype. Current available data does not allow clarification as to whether the neuroendocrine component arises through trans-differentiation of the non-neuroendocrine one or the two components develop independently. Either way, these findings open new avenues for the exploration of targeted treatments and immunotherapies with already proven activity in the treatment of GEP adenocarcinomas.

In conclusion, the MiNEN is likely an underestimated disease, due to the controversies relating to its definition, the limited diagnostic ability of biopsies, and the lack of awareness of this diagnosis within the scientific community (suggested by the absence of clinical trials enrolling patients with this diagnosis, and the minimal referencing by major international oncology societies). To increase the likelihood of diagnosing MiNEN, core biopsies should be sought when a surgical sample is not available, and analysed by pathologists with expertise in neuroendocrine neoplasms.

Because of the low quality of the evidence collected, it is very difficult to formulate recommendations on the best management of patients with an MiNEN diagnosis. Therefore, newly diagnosed patients with MiNENs should be discussed within multidisciplinary meetings and the treatment strategy should be planned on the basis of the most aggressive and/or predominant component in the diagnostic sample. Following the standard practice for their pure counterparts is entirely appropriate given that randomised studies are unlikely to be feasible in this patient group. Furthermore, since only one of the two components is present in most distant metastatic sites, the collection of a second tumour sample is advisable to optimise the management and guide the choice of systemic treatment in the following scenarios; (1) in the presence of synchronous distant metastases when the original sample is from the primary tumour, (2) on metastatic recurrence of a previously resected MiNEN, and (3) on development of new/rapidly growing metastatic lesions while on treatment, in the setting of otherwise stable disease. The advent of liquid biopsies may aid in delivering more customised treatments for these diseases. Genomic profiling of tumour or blood samples of patients diagnosed with an MiNEN should be encouraged, with a view to widening the knowledge of the biology of this disease and possibly offering those patients participation in prospective early phase or basket type/umbrella clinical trials.

Supplementary Materials: The following are available online at http://www.mdpi.com/2077-0383/9/1/273/s1. Table S1. Survival outcomes of patients with a diagnosis of mixed neuroendocrine non-neuroendocrine neoplasms in retrospective studies where median survival estimates by Kaplan–Meier analysis were not reached. Table S2. Comparison of survival outcomes of mixed neuroendocrine non-neuroendocrine neoplasms with survival outcomes of other neoplasms from the same sites of origin.

Author Contributions: M.F., B.N.: literature search, data analysis, and manuscript writing. M.G.M.: conception of the idea and design of the review, manuscript writing, review and proof-reading, and approval of the final version. B.C., R.A.H., A.L., and J.W.V.: manuscript review, proof-reading, and approval of the final version. All authors have read and agreed to the published version of the manuscript.

Funding: This research did not receive a specific grant from funding agencies in the public, commercial, or non-profit sectors.

Conflicts of Interest: The authors declare no conflict of interest.

References

1. Volante, M.; Rindi, G.; Papotti, M. The grey zone between pure (neuro)endocrine and non-(neuro)endocrine tumours: A comment on concepts and classification of mixed exocrine-endocrine neoplasms. *Virchows Arch.* **2006**, *449*, 499–506. [CrossRef] [PubMed]
2. La Rosa, S.; Sessa, F.; Uccella, S. Mixed Neuroendocrine-Nonneuroendocrine Neoplasms (MiNENs): Unifying the Concept of a Heterogeneous Group of Neoplasms. *Endocr. Pathol.* **2016**, *27*, 284–311. [CrossRef]

3. Lewin, K. Carcinoid tumors and the mixed (composite) glandular-endocrine cell carcinomas. *Am. J. Surg. Pathol.* **1987**, *11* (Suppl. 1), 71–86. [CrossRef] [PubMed]
4. Bosman, F.T.; Carneiro, F.; Hruban, R.H.; Theise, N.D. *WHO Classification of Tumours of the Digestive System*, 4th ed.; International Agency for Research on Cancer (IARC): Lyon, France, 2010.
5. Lloyd, R.V.; Osamura, R.Y.; Klöppel, G.; Rosai, J. *Who Classification of Tumours of Endocrine Organs*, 4th ed.; International Agency for Research on Cancer (IARC): Lyon, France, 2017.
6. WHO Classification of Tumours Editorial Board. *WHO Classification of Tumours. Digestive System Tumours*, 5th ed.; International Agency for Research on Cancer (IARC): Lyon, France, 2019.
7. La Rosa, S.; Marando, A.; Sessa, F.; Capella, C. Mixed Adenoneuroendocrine Carcinomas (MANECs) of the Gastrointestinal Tract: An Update. *Cancers* **2012**, *4*, 11–30. [CrossRef]
8. Garcia-Carbonero, R.; Sorbye, H.; Baudin, E.; Raymond, E.; Wiedenmann, B.; Niederle, B.; Sedlackova, E.; Toumpanakis, C.; Anlauf, M.; Cwikla, J.B.; et al. ENETS Consensus Guidelines for High-Grade Gastroenteropancreatic Neuroendocrine Tumors and Neuroendocrine Carcinomas. *Neuroendocrinology* **2016**, *103*, 186–194. [CrossRef] [PubMed]
9. Bazerbachi, F.; Kermanshahi, T.R.; Monteiro, C. Early precursor of mixed endocrine-exocrine tumors of the gastrointestinal tract: Histologic and molecular correlations. *Ochsner J.* **2015**, *15*, 97–101. [PubMed]
10. Girardi, D.M.; Silva, A.C.B.; Rêgo, J.F.M.; Coudry, R.A.; Riechelmann, R.P. Unraveling molecular pathways of poorly differentiated neuroendocrine carcinomas of the gastroenteropancreatic system: A systematic review. *Cancer Treat. Rev.* **2017**, *56*, 28–35. [CrossRef]
11. Golombek, T.; Henker, R.; Rehak, M.; Quäschling, U.; Lordick, F.; Knödler, M. A Rare Case of Mixed Adenoneuroendocrine Carcinoma (MANEC) of the Gastroesophageal Junction with HER2/neu Overexpression and Distinct Orbital and Optic Nerve Toxicity after Intravenous Administration of Cisplatin. *Oncol. Res. Treat.* **2019**, *42*, 123–127. [CrossRef] [PubMed]
12. Kubo, K.; Kimura, N.; Mabe, K.; Nishimura, Y.; Kato, M. Synchronous Triple Gastric Cancer Incorporating Mixed Adenocarcinoma and Neuroendocrine Tumor Completely Resected with Endoscopic Submucosal Dissection. *Intern. Med.* **2018**, *57*, 2951–2955. [CrossRef]
13. Lin, Z.; Chen, J.; Guo, Y. Efficacy of XELOX adjuvant chemotherapy for gastric mixed adenoneuroendocrine carcinoma: A case report. *Medicine (Baltimore)* **2019**, *98*, e16000. [CrossRef]
14. Kim, K.H.; Lee, H.J.; Lee, S.H.; Hwang, S.H. Mixed adenoneuroendocrine carcinoma in the stomach: A case report with a literature review. *Ann. Surg. Treat. Res.* **2018**, *94*, 270–273. [CrossRef] [PubMed]
15. Ochiai, T.; Ominami, M.; Nagami, Y.; Fukunaga, S.; Toyokawa, T.; Yamagami, H.; Tanigawa, T.; Watanabe, T.; Ohira, M.; Ohsawa, M.; et al. Lymph Node Metastasis of Mixed Adenoneuroendocrine Carcinoma after Curative Resection Using the Expanded Criteria for Early Gastric Cancer. *Intern. Med.* **2018**, *57*, 2837–2842. [CrossRef] [PubMed]
16. Yang, G.; Li, D.; Zheng, F.; Yang, L. Long-term disease free survival of gastric mixed adenoneuroendocrine carcinoma treated with multimodality therapy: A case report. *Mol. Clin. Oncol.* **2018**, *8*, 653–656. [CrossRef] [PubMed]
17. Pastorello, R.G.; de Macedo, M.P.; da Costa Junior, W.L.; Begnami, M.D.F.S. Gastric Pouch Mixed Adenoneuroendocrine Carcinoma with a Mixed Adenocarcinoma Component after Roux-en-Y Gastric Bypass. *J. Investig. Med. High Impact Case Rep.* **2017**, *5*, 2324709617740908. [CrossRef] [PubMed]
18. Shimizu, A.; Takahashi, T.; Kushima, R.; Sentani, K.; Yasui, W.; Matsuno, Y. An extremely rare case of Epstein-Barr virus-associated gastric carcinoma with differentiation to neuroendocrine carcinoma. *Pathol. Int.* **2018**, *68*, 41–46. [CrossRef] [PubMed]
19. Tang, Q.; Zhou, Z.; Chen, J.; Di, M.; Ji, J.; Yuan, W.; Liu, Z.; Wu, L.; Zhang, X.; Li, K.; et al. Correlation of metastasis characteristics with prognosis in gastric mixed adenoneuroendocrine carcinoma: Two case reports. *Medicine (Baltimore)* **2017**, *96*, e9189. [CrossRef]
20. Kheiri, B.; Osman, M.; Congdon, D.; Bachuwa, G. A rare case of gastric mixed adenoneuroendocrine carcinoma (MANEC) with gastric Helicobacter pylori-negative mucosa-associated lymphoid tissue (MALT) lymphoma. *BMJ Case Rep.* **2017**, *2017*. [CrossRef]
21. Nassereddine, H.; Poté, N.; Théou-Anton, N.; Lamoureux, G.; Fléjou, J.F.; Couvelard, A. A gastric MANEC with an adenocarcinoma of fundic-gland type as exocrine component. *Virchows Arch.* **2017**, *471*, 673–678. [CrossRef]

22. Pham, Q.D.; Mori, I.; Osamura, R.Y. A Case Report: Gastric Mixed Neuroendocrine-Nonneuroendocrine Neoplasm with Aggressive Neuroendocrine Component. *Case Rep. Pathol.* **2017**, *2017*, 9871687. [CrossRef]
23. Cazzo, E.; de Saito, H.P. Mixed adenoneuroendocrine carcinoma of the gastric stump following Billroth II gastrectomy: Case report and review of the literature. *Sao Paulo Med. J.* **2016**, *134*, 84–87. [CrossRef]
24. De Luca-Johnson, J.; Zenali, M. A Previously Undescribed Presentation of Mixed Adenoneuroendocrine Carcinoma. *Case Rep. Pathol.* **2016**, *2016*, 9063634. [CrossRef] [PubMed]
25. Yamasaki, Y.; Nasu, J.; Miura, K.; Kono, Y.; Kanzaki, H.; Hori, K.; Tanaka, T.; Kita, M.; Tsuzuki, T.; Matsubara, M.; et al. Intramucosal gastric mixed adenoneuroendocrine carcinoma completely resected with endoscopic submucosal dissection. *Intern. Med.* **2015**, *54*, 917–920. [CrossRef] [PubMed]
26. Fukuba, N.; Yuki, T.; Ishihara, S.; Sonoyama, H.; Tada, Y.; Kusunoki, R.; Oka, A.; Oshima, N.; Moriyama, I.; Kawashima, K.; et al. Gastric mixed adenoneuroendocrine carcinoma with a good prognosis. *Intern. Med.* **2014**, *53*, 2585–2588. [CrossRef] [PubMed]
27. Taguchi, J.; Shinozaki, K.; Baba, S.; Kurogi, J.; Nakane, T.; Kinoshita, Y.; Ishii, K.; Ueno, T.; Torimura, T.; Yano, H. A resected case of neuroendocrine carcinoma of the stomach with unusual lymph node metastasis. *Med. Mol. Morphol.* **2016**, *49*, 34–41. [CrossRef] [PubMed]
28. Zecchini, R.; Azzolini, F.; Cecinato, P.; Iori, V.; De Marco, L.; Zanelli, M.; Parmeggiani, F.; Cavina, M.; Sereni, G.; Tioli, C.; et al. Sassatelli, R. A rare case of mixed adeno-neuroendocrine gastric carcinoma (MANEC) associated to autoimmune metaplastic atrophic gastritis (AMAG). *Dig. Liver Dis.* **2016**, *48* (Suppl. 2), e148. [CrossRef]
29. Farooq, F.; Zarrabi, K.; Sweeney, K.; Kim, J.; Bandovic, J.; Patel, C.; Choi, M. Multiregion Comprehensive Genomic Profiling of a Gastric Mixed Neuroendocrine-Nonneuroendocrine Neoplasm with Trilineage Differentiation. *J. Gastric Cancer* **2018**, *18*, 200–207. [CrossRef] [PubMed]
30. Fujita, Y.; Uesugi, N.; Sugimoto, R.; Eizuka, M.; Matsumoto, T.; Sugai, T. Gastric mixed neuroendocrine-non-neuroendocrine neoplasm (MiNEN) with pancreatic acinar differentiation: A case report. *Diagn. Pathol.* **2019**, *14*, 38. [CrossRef]
31. Zhang, W.; Xiao, W.; Ma, H.; Sun, M.; Chen, H.; Zheng, S. Neuroendocrine liver metastasis in gastric mixed adenoneuroendocrine carcinoma with trilineage cell differentiation: A case report. *Int. J. Clin. Exp. Pathol.* **2014**, *7*, 6333–6338.
32. Juanmartinena, J.F.; Fernández-Urién, I.; Córdoba, A.; Miranda, C.; Borda, A. Mixed adenoneuroendocrine carcinoma (MANEC) of the gastroesophageal junction: A case report and review of the literature. *Rev. Esp. Enferm. Dig.* **2017**, *109*, 160–162. [CrossRef]
33. Yamamoto, M.; Ozawa, S.; Koyanagi, K.; Oguma, J.; Kazuno, A.; Ninomiya, Y.; Yatabe, K.; Hatanaka, K. Mixed adenoneuroendocrine carcinoma of the esophagogastric junction: A case report. *Surg. Case Rep.* **2018**, *4*, 56. [CrossRef]
34. Uda, S.; Makuuchi, H.; Nitta, M.; Kazuno, A.; Yamamoto, S.; Nishi, T.; Chino, O.; Shimada, H.; Ozawa, S. A case of mixed adenoneuroendcrine carcinoma (MANEC) of the esophagogastric junction. *Dis. Esophagus* **2014**, *27*, P2.14.22.
35. Yuan, W.; Liu, Z.; Lei, W.; Sun, L.; Yang, H.; Wang, Y.; Ramdas, S.; Dong, X.; Xu, R.; Cai, H.; et al. Mutation landscape and intra-tumor heterogeneity of two MANECs of the esophagus revealed by multi-region sequencing. *Oncotarget* **2017**, *8*, 69610–69621. [PubMed]
36. Imaoka, K.; Fukuda, S.; Tazawa, H.; Kuga, Y.; Mochizuki, T.; Hirata. Y.; Fujisaki, S.; Takahashi, M.; Nishida, T.; Sakimoto, H. A mixed adenoneuroendocrine carcinoma of the pancreas: A case report. *Surg. Case Rep.* **2016**, *2*, 133. [CrossRef] [PubMed]
37. Lee, L.; Bajor-Dattilo, E.B.; Das, K. Metastatic mixed acinar-neuroendocrine carcinoma of the pancreas to the liver: A cytopathology case report with review of the literature. *Diagn. Cytopathol.* **2013**, *41*, 164–170. [CrossRef]
38. Mahansaria, S.S.; Agrawal, N.; Arora, A.; Bihari, C.; Appukuttan, M.; Chattopadhyay, T.K. Ampullary Mixed Adenoneuroendocrine Carcinoma: Surprise Histology, Familiar Management. *Int. J. Surg. Pathol.* **2017**, *25*, 585–591. [CrossRef]
39. Zhang, L.; Yang, Z.; Chen, Q.; Li, M.; Zhu, X.; Wan, D.; Xie, H.; Zheng, S. Mixed adenoendocrine carcinoma in the extrahepatic biliary tract: A case report and literature review. *Oncol. Lett.* **2019**, *18*, 1585–1596. [CrossRef]

40. Skalicky, A.; Vištejnová, L.; Dubová, M.; Malkus, T.; Skalický, T.; Troup, O. Mixed neuroendocrine-non-neuroendocrine carcinoma of gallbladder: Case report. *World J. Surg. Oncol.* **2019**, *17*, 55. [CrossRef]
41. Yoshioka, S.; Ebisu, Y.; Ishida, M.; Uemura, Y.; Yanagimoto, H.; Satoi, S.; Tsuta, K. Cytological features of mixed adenoneuroendocrine carcinoma of the ampulla of Vater: A case report with immunocytochemical analyses. *Diagn. Cytopathol.* **2018**, *46*, 540–546. [CrossRef]
42. Komo, T.; Kohashi, T.; Nakashima, A.; Ohmori, I.; Hihara, J.; Mukaida, H.; Kaneko, M.; Hirabayashi, N. Mixed adenoneuroendocrine carcinoma of the distal bile duct: A case report. *Int. J. Surg. Case Rep.* **2017**, *39*, 203–207. [CrossRef]
43. Izumo, W.; Higuchi, R.; Yazawa, T.; Uemura, S.; Matsunaga, Y.; Shiihara, M.; Furukawa, T.; Yamamoto, M. A long-term recurrence-free survival of a patient with the mixed adeno-neuroendocrine bile duct carcinoma: A case report and review of the literature. *Int. J. Surg. Case Rep.* **2017**, *39*, 43–50. [CrossRef]
44. Takemoto, Y.K.; Abe, T.; Amano, H.; Hanada, K.; Okazaki, A.; Minami, T.; Kobayashi, T.; Nakahara, M.; Yonehara, S.; Ohdan, H.; et al. Mixed adenoneuroendocrine carcinoma derived from the cystic duct: A case report. *Int. J. Surg. Case Rep.* **2017**, *39*, 29–33. [CrossRef] [PubMed]
45. Huang, Z.; Xiao, W.D.; Li, Y.; Huang, S.; Cai, J.; Ao, J. Mixed adenoneuroendocrine carcinoma of the ampulla: Two case reports. *World J. Gastroenterol.* **2015**, *21*, 2254–2259. [CrossRef] [PubMed]
46. Meguro, Y.; Fukushima, N.; Koizumi, M.; Kasahara, N.; Hydo, M.; Morishima, K.; Sata, N.; Lefor, A.T.; Yasuda, Y. A case of mixed adenoneuroendocrine carcinoma of the gallbladder arising from an intracystic papillary neoplasm associated with pancreaticobiliary maljunction. *Pathol. Int.* **2014**, *64*, 465–471. [CrossRef] [PubMed]
47. Zhang, L.; DeMay, R.M. Cytological features of mixed adenoneuroendocrine carcinoma of the ampulla: Two case reports with review of literature. *Diagn. Cytopathol.* **2014**, *42*, 1075–1084. [CrossRef] [PubMed]
48. Shintaku, M.; Kataoka, K.; Kawabata, K. Mixed adenoneuroendocrine carcinoma of the gallbladder with squamous cell carcinomatous and osteosarcomatous differentiation: Report of a case. *Pathol. Int.* **2013**, *63*, 113–119. [CrossRef]
49. Song, W.; Chen, W.; Zhang, S.; Peng, J.; He, Y. Successful treatment of gallbladder mixed adenoneuroendocrine carcinoma with neo-adjuvant chemotherapy. *Diagn. Pathol.* **2012**, *7*, 163. [CrossRef]
50. Sato, O.; Tsuchikawa, T.; Yamada, T.; Sato, D.; Nakanishi, Y.; Asano, T.; Noji, T.; Yo, K.; Ebihara, Y.; Murakami, S.; et al. Metastatic mixed adenoneuroendocrine carcinoma of the liver successfully resected by hepatic trisectionectomy following chemotherapy: A case report. *Clin. Case Rep.* **2019**, *7*, 491–496.
51. Silva, J.R.D.; Pinho, R.T.; Furtado, A. A case of a mixed adenoneuroendocrine tumor of the colon. *Rev. Esp. Enferm. Dig.* **2017**, *109*, 673. [CrossRef]
52. Carboni, F.; Valle, M.; Russo, A. Mixed adenoneuroendocrine carcinoma of the cecum. *Clin. Res. Hepatol. Gastroenterol.* **2019**, *43*, 627–629. [CrossRef]
53. Cherbanyk, F.; Gassend, J.L.; Dimitrief, M.; Andrejevic-Blant, S.; Martinet, O.; Pezzetta, E. A Rare Type of Colorectal Cancer: Mixed Adeno-Neuroendocrine Carcinoma (MANEC). *Chirurgia (Bucharest)* **2017**, *112*, 152–156. [CrossRef]
54. Morais, M.; Pinho, A.C.; Marques, A.; Lopes, J.; Duarte, A.; da Silva, P.C.; Lopes, J.M.; Maia, J.C. Mixed Adenoneuroendocrine Carcinoma Causing Colonic Intussusception. *Case Rep. Surg.* **2016**, *2016*, 7684364. [PubMed]
55. Tagai, N.; Goi, T.; Morikawa, M.; Kurebayashi, H.; Kato, S.; Fujimoto, D.; Koneri, K.; Murakami, M.; Hirono, Y.; Noriki, S.; et al. Favorable response of colonic mixed adenoneuroendocrine carcinoma to streptozocin monotherapy. *Int. Cancer Conf. J.* **2017**, *6*, 175–179. [CrossRef] [PubMed]
56. Gurzu, S.; Kadar, Z.; Bara, T.; Bara, T., Jr.; Tamasi, A.; Azamfirei, L.; Jung, I. Mixed adenoneuroendocrine carcinoma of gastrointestinal tract: Report of two cases. *World J. Gastroenterol.* **2015**, *21*, 1329–1333. [CrossRef] [PubMed]
57. Minaya-Bravo, A.M.; Garcia Mahillo, J.C.; Mendoza Moreno, F.; Noguelares Fraguas, F.; Granell, J. Large cell neuroendocrine—Adenocarcinona mixed tumour of colon: Collision tumour with peculiar behaviour. What do we know about these tumours? *Ann. Med. Surg. (Lond.)* **2015**, *4*, 399–403.
58. Vanacker, L.; Smeets, D.; Hoorens, A.; Teugels, E.; Algaba, R.; Dehou, M.F.; De Becker, A.; Lambrechts, D.; De Greve, J. Mixed adenoneuroendocrine carcinoma of the colon: Molecular pathogenesis and treatment. *Anticancer Res.* **2014**, *34*, 5517–5521.

59. Ito, H.; Kudo, A.; Matsumura, S.; Ban, D.; Irie, T.; Ochiai, T.; Nakamura, N.; Tanaka, S.; Tanabe, M. Mixed adenoneuroendocrine carcinoma of the colon progressed rapidly after hepatic rupture: Report of a case. *Int. Surg.* **2014**, *99*, 40–44. [CrossRef]
60. Khudiakov, A.; Al-Sadawi, M.; Qin, J.; Haddadin, M.; Soroka, S.; Hartt, A.; Soni, L.; Arora, S.; McFarlane, S.I. Rare Case of Rectal Mixed Adeno-Neuroendocrine Carcinoma. *Am. J. Med. Case Rep.* **2019**, *7*, 117–120. [CrossRef]
61. Yamauchi, H.; Sakurai, S.; Tsukagoshi, R.; Suzuki, M.; Tabe, Y.; Fukasawa, T.; Kiriyama, S.; Fukuchi, M.; Naitoh, H.; Kuwano, H. A case of very well-differentiated adenocarcinoma with carcinoid tumor in the ascending colon. *Int. Surg.* **2014**, *99*, 132–136.
62. Semrau, S.; Agaimy, A.; Pavel, M.; Lubgan, D.; Schmidt, D.; Cavallaro, A.; Golcher, H.; Grützmann, R.; Fietkau, R. Long-term control with chemoradiation of initially metastatic mixed adenoneuroendocrine carcinoma of the rectum: A case report. *J. Med. Case Rep.* **2019**, *13*, 82. [PubMed]
63. Constantinou, P.; Karagkounis, G.; Kazamias, G.; Taliadoros, A.; Poullou, C.; Vourlakou, C. Metastatic Mixed Mdenoneuroendocrine Carcinomas (MANECs) of the colorectum: Two cases. *Virchows Arch.* **2015**, *467*, S184–S185.
64. Quaas, A.; Waldschmidt, D.; Alakus, H.; Zander, T.; Heydt, C.; Goeser, T.; Daheim, M.; Kasper, P.; Plum, P.; Bruns, C.; et al. Therapy susceptible germline-related BRCA 1-mutation in a case of metastasized mixed adeno-neuroendocrine carcinoma (MANEC) of the small bowel. *BMC Gastroenterol.* **2018**, *18*, 75. [CrossRef] [PubMed]
65. Steel, C.J.; Hostetler, V.; Dunn, D. A case of hyperfunctioning pancreatic mixed adenoneuroendocrine carcinoma (MANEC) arising from ectopic pancreatic tissue in the liver. *Radiol. Case Rep.* **2014**, *9*, 1011. [CrossRef] [PubMed]
66. Mehrvarz Sarshekeh, A.; Advani, S.; Patel, M.R.; Dasari, A. Prognostic validity of AJCC staging system in neuroendocrine tumors of the appendix. *Ann. Oncol.* **2016**, *27* (Suppl. 6).
67. Melchior, L.C.; Willemoe, G.L.; Garbyal, R.S.; Langer, S.W.; Knigge, U.; Federspiel, B. Next generation sequencing of 294 neuroendocrine g3 and mixed neuroendocrine and non-neuroendocrine neoplasms identifies molecular profile linked to the site of the primary and tumor composition. *Neuroendocrinology* **2019**, *108* (Suppl. 1), 31.
68. Pop, G.; Popp, C.G.; Nichita, L.; Gramada, E.; Sticlaru, L.C.; Dutulescu, S.; Michire-Stefana, A.D.; Stanga, P.I.; Mastalier, B.; Staniceanu, F. Pancreatic mixed adeno-neuroendocrine carcinomas (MANECs)-report of a series of cases. *Virchows Arch.* **2016**, *469*, PS-05-026.
69. Brathwaite, S.; Rock, J.; Yearsley, M.M.; Bekaii-Saab, T.; Wei, L.; Frankel, W.L.; Hays, J.; Wu, C.; Abdel-Misih, S. Mixed Adeno-neuroendocrine Carcinoma: An Aggressive Clinical Entity. *Ann. Surg. Oncol.* **2016**, *23*, 2281–2286. [CrossRef]
70. Brathwaite, S.; Yearsley, M.M.; Bekaii-Saab, T.; Wei, L.; Schmidt, C.R.; Dillhoff, M.E.; Frankel, W.L.; Hays, J.; Wu, C.; Abdel-Misih, S. Appendiceal Mixed Adeno-Neuroendocrine Carcinoma: A Population-Based Study of the Surveillance, Epidemiology, and End Results Registry. *Front. Oncol.* **2016**, *6*, 148. [CrossRef]
71. Yang, H.-M.; Schaaf, C.; Schaeffer, D.; Vieth, M.; Veits, L.; Geddert, H.; Jung, A.; Kirchner, T.; Horst, D. Molecular analysis of mixed adenoneuroendocrine carcinomas (MANEC) signifies a common clonal origin of adeno and neuroendocrine components. *Lab. Investig.* **2015**, *95*, 199A.
72. Basturk, O.; Adsay, V.; Hruban, R.H.; Yang, Z.; Giordano, T.J.; Shi, C.; Saka, B.; Klimstra, D.S. Pancreatic acinar cell carcinomas with prominent neuroendocrine differentiation: Clinicopathologic analysis of a distinct and diagnostically challenging neoplasm. *Lab. Investig.* **2014**, *94*, 447A.
73. Dulskas, A.; Pilvelis, A. Oncologic outcome of mixed adenoneuroendocrine carcinoma (MANEC): A single center case series. *Eur. J. Surg. Oncol.* **2019**, *46*, 105–107. [CrossRef]
74. Duzkoylu, Y.; Aras, O.; Bostancı, E.B.; Keklik Temuçin, T.; Ulaş, M. Mixed Adeno-Neuroendocrine Carcinoma; Case Series of Ten Patients with Review of the Literature. *Balkan Med. J.* **2018**, *35*, 263–267. [CrossRef]
75. Apostolidis, L.; Haag, G.M.; Jager, D.; Winkler, E.C.; Bergmann, F. Treatment outcomes of patients with mixed neuroendocrine non-neuroendocrine neoplasms (MINEN). *Neuroendocrinology* **2018**, *106*, 56.
76. Bu, S.; Ding, D.; Wang, X.; Fan, R.; Xu, J.; Chen, Y.; Liu, H. The clinical characteristics and prognosis of 73 patients with Nonfunctional Gastroenteropancreatic neuroendocrine neoplasm: A 10-year retrospective study of a single center. *Clin. Pract.* **2017**, *14*, 198–203. [CrossRef]

77. Lee, S.M.; Broaddus, R.; Singh, R.; Luthra, R.; Chen, H. Mutation profile of colorectal neuroendocrine neoplasm. *Lab. Investig.* **2016**, *96*, 182A.
78. Kolasinska-Cwikla, A.D.; Lewczuk, A.; Cichocki, A.; Maciejkiewicz, K.; Nowicka, E.; Roszkowska-Purska, K.; Jodkiewicz, Z.; Tenderenda, M.; C'wikła, J.B. Neuroendocrine carcinomas of the colorectal origin—Polish experience. *Ann. Oncol.* **2016**, *27* (Suppl. 6). [CrossRef]
79. Jesinghaus, M.; Konukiewitz, B.; Keller, G.; Kloor, M.; Steiger, K.; Reiche, M.; Penzel, R.; Endris, V.; Arseni, R.; Hermann, G.; et al. Colorectal mixed adenoneuroendocrine carcinomas and neuroendocrine carcinomas are genetically closely related to colorectal adenocarcinomas. *Mod. Pathol.* **2017**, *30*, 610–619. [CrossRef] [PubMed]
80. Komatsubara, T.; Koinuma, K.; Miyakura, Y.; Horie, H.; Morimoto, M.; Ito, H.; Lefor, A.K.; Sata, N.; Fukushima, N. Endocrine cell carcinomas of the colon and rectum: A clinicopathological evaluation. *Clin. J. Gastroenterol.* **2016**, *9*, 1–6. [CrossRef]
81. La Rosa, S.; Bernasconi, B.; Vanoli, A.; Sciarra, A.; Notohara, K.; Albarello, L.; Casnedi, S.; Billo, P.; Zhang, L.; Tibiletti, M.G.; et al. c-MYC amplification and c-myc protein expression in pancreatic acinar cell carcinomas. New insights into the molecular signature of these rare cancers. *Virchows Arch.* **2018**, *473*, 435–441. [CrossRef]
82. La Rosa, S.; Uccella, S.; Molinari, F.; Savio, A.; Mete, O.; Vanoli, A.; Maragliano, R.; Frattini, M.; Mazzucchelli, L.; Sessa, F.; et al. Mixed Adenoma Well-differentiated Neuroendocrine Tumor (MANET) of the Digestive System: An Indolent Subtype of Mixed Neuroendocrine-NonNeuroendocrine Neoplasm (MiNEN). *Am. J. Surg. Pathol.* **2018**, *42*, 1503–1512. [CrossRef]
83. Lim, S.M.; Kim, H.; Kang, B.; Kim, H.S.; Rha, S.Y.; Noh, S.H.; Hyung, W.J.; Cheong, J.H.; Kim, H.I.; Chung, H.C.; et al. Prognostic value of (18)F-fluorodeoxyglucose positron emission tomography in patients with gastric neuroendocrine carcinoma and mixed adenoneuroendocrine carcinoma. *Ann. Nucl. Med.* **2016**, *30*, 279–286. [CrossRef]
84. Frizziero, M.; Wang, X.; Chakrabarty, B.; Childs, A.; Luong, L.V.; Walter, T.; Elshafie, M.; Shah, T.; Fulford, P.; Minicozzi, A.; et al. Mixed adeno-neuroendocrine carcinoma (MANEC) of the gastroenteropancreatic (GEP) tract: A multicentre retrospective study. *Ann. Oncol.* **2017**, *28* (Suppl. 5). [CrossRef]
85. Milione, M.; Maisonneuve, P.; Pellegrinelli, A.; Grillo, F.; Albarello, L.; Spaggiari, P.; Vanoli, A.; Tagliabue, G.; Pisa, E.; Messerini, L.; et al. Ki67 proliferative index of the neuroendocrine component drives MANEC prognosis. *Endocr. Relat. Cancer* **2018**, *25*, 583–593. [CrossRef] [PubMed]
86. Nie, L.; Li, M.; He, X.; Feng, A.; Wu, H.; Fan, X. Gastric mixed adenoneuroendocrine carcinoma: Correlation of histologic characteristics with prognosis. *Ann. Diagn. Pathol.* **2016**, *25*, 48–53. [CrossRef] [PubMed]
87. Schimmack, S.; Weber, T.; Bergmann, F.; Hinz, U.; Nießen, A.; Hackert, T.; Büchler, M.W.; Strobel, O. Mixed exocrine-endocrine neoplasms of the pancreas. *Langenbecks Arch. Surg.* **2017**, *402*, 1136.
88. Park, J.Y.; Ryu, M.H.; Park, Y.S.; Park, H.J.; Ryoo, B.Y.; Kim, M.G.; Yook, J.H.; Kim, B.S.; Kang, Y.K. Prognostic significance of neuroendocrine components in gastric carcinomas. *Eur. J. Cancer* **2014**, *50*, 2802–2809. [CrossRef] [PubMed]
89. Olevian, D.; Harris, B.; Nikiforova, M.; Kuan, S.-F.; Pai, R. Clinicopathologic analysis of colorectal carcinoma with high-grade neuroendocrine differentiation: Identification of a unique subtype with mixed large cell neuroendocrine carcinoma/signet ring cell adenocarcinoma with frequent BRAF mutation and poor overall survival. *Lab. Investig.* **2015**, *95*, 182A.
90. Spada, F.; Milione, M.; Maisonneuve, P.; Prinzi, N.; Smiroldo, V.; Bolzacchini, E.; Carnaghi, C.; La Rosa, S.; Cappella, C.; Sessa, F.; et al. An Italian Multicenter Study in Patients with Advanced Mixed AdenoNeuroendocrine Carcinomas (MANECs) of the Gastro-Entero-Pancreatic Tract Treated with Chemotherapy. *Neuroendocrinology* **2019**, *108*, 190.
91. Bongiovanni, M.; Molinari, F.; Uccella, S.; Savio, A.; Sessa, F.; La Rosa, S. Mixed Adenoma-Well Differentiated Neuroendocrine Tumors (MANETs) of the Colon. Clinico-Pathologic and Molecular Analysis of 6 Cases of a Rare and Recently Recognized Entity. *Lab. Investig.* **2017**, *97*, 145A.
92. Sahnane, N.; Furlan, D.; Monti, M.; Romualdi, C.; Vanoli, A.; Vicari, E.; Solcia, E.; Capella, C.; Sessa, F.; La Rosa, S. Microsatellite unstable gastrointestinal neuroendocrine carcinomas: A new clinicopathologic entity. *Endocr. Relat. Cancer* **2015**, *22*, 35–45. [CrossRef]

93. Scardoni, M.; Vittoria, E.; Volante, M.; Rusev, B.; Bersani, S.; Mafficini, A.; Gottardi, M.; Giandomenico, V.; Malleo, G.; Butturini, G.; et al. Mixed adenoneuroendocrine carcinomas of the gastrointestinal tract: Targeted next-generation sequencing suggests a monoclonal origin of the two components. *Neuroendocrinology* **2014**, *100*, 310–316. [CrossRef]
94. Shen, C.; Chen, H.; Chen, H.; Yin, Y.; Han, L.; Chen, J.; Tang, S.; Yin, X.; Zhou, Z.; Zhang, B.; et al. Surgical treatment and prognosis of gastric neuroendocrine neoplasms: A single-center experience. *BMC Gastroenterol.* **2016**, *16*, 111. [CrossRef]
95. Sinha, N.; Gaston, D.; Manders, D.; Goudie, M.; Matsuoka, M.; Xie, T.; Huang, W.Y. Characterization of genome-wide copy number aberrations in colonic mixed adenoneuroendocrine carcinoma and neuroendocrine carcinoma reveals recurrent amplification of PTGER4 and MYC genes. *Hum. Pathol.* **2018**, *73*, 16–25. [CrossRef] [PubMed]
96. van der Veen, A.; Seesing, M.F.; Wijnhoven, B.P.L.; de Steur, W.O.; van Berge Henegouwen, M.I.; Rosman, C.; van Sandick, J.W.; Mook, S.; Haj Mohammad, N.; Ruurda, J.P.; et al. Management of resectable esophageal and gastric (mixed adeno) neuroendocrine carcinoma: A nationwide cohort study. *Eur. J. Surg. Oncol.* **2018**, *44*, 1955–1962. [CrossRef] [PubMed]
97. Woischke, C.; Schaaf, C.W.; Yang, H.M.; Vieth, M.; Veits, L.; Geddert, H.; Märkl, B.; Stömmer, P.; Schaeffer, D.F.; Frölich, M.; et al. In-depth mutational analyses of colorectal neuroendocrine carcinomas with adenoma or adenocarcinoma components. *Mod. Pathol.* **2017**, *30*, 95–103. [CrossRef] [PubMed]
98. Yang, M.; Tan, C.L.; Zhang, Y.; Ke, N.W.; Zeng, L.; Li, A.; Zhang, H.; Xiong, J.J.; Guo, Z.H.; Tian, B.L.; et al. B Applications of a novel tumor-grading-metastasis staging system for pancreatic neuroendocrine tumors: An analysis of surgical patients from a Chinese institution. *Medicine (Baltimore)* **2016**, *95*, e4213. [CrossRef] [PubMed]
99. Yin, X.N.; Shen, C.Y.; Yin, Y.Q.; Chen, H.J.; Chen, H.N.; Yin, Y.; Han, L.Y.; Chen, J.J.; Tang, S.M.; Chen, Z.X.; et al. Prognoses in patients with primary gastrointestinal neuroendocrine neoplasms based on the proposed new classification scheme. *Asia Pac. J. Clin. Oncol.* **2018**, *14*, e37–e44. [CrossRef]
100. Zhang, P.; Wang, W.; Lu, M.; Zeng, C.; Chen, J.; Li, E.; Tan, H.; Wang, W.; Yu, X.; Tang, Q.; et al. Clinicopathological features and outcome for neuroendocrine neoplasms of gastroesophageal junction: A population-based study. *Cancer Med.* **2018**, *7*, 4361–4370. [CrossRef]
101. Zheng, Z.; Chen, C.; Li, B.; Liu, H.; Zhou, L.; Zhang, H.; Zheng, C.; He, X.; Liu, W.; Hong, T.; et al. Biliary Neuroendocrine Neoplasms: Clinical Profiles, Management, and Analysis of Prognostic Factors. *Front. Oncol.* **2019**, *9*, 38. [CrossRef]
102. Iannuccelli, M.; Micarelli, E.; Surdo, P.L.; Palma, A.; Perfetto, L.; Rozzo, I.; Castagnoli, L.; Licata, L.; Cesareni, G. CancerGeneNet: Linking driver genes to cancer hallmarks. *Nucleic Acids Res.* **2019**, *48*, D416–D421. [CrossRef]

© 2020 by the authors. Licensee MDPI, Basel, Switzerland. This article is an open access article distributed under the terms and conditions of the Creative Commons Attribution (CC BY) license (http://creativecommons.org/licenses/by/4.0/).

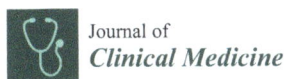

Review

Follow-Up Recommendations after Curative Resection of Well-Differentiated Neuroendocrine Tumours: Review of Current Evidence and Clinical Practice

Angela Lamarca [1,2,*], Hamish Clouston [3], Jorge Barriuso [1,2], Mairéad G McNamara [1,2], Melissa Frizziero [1,2], Was Mansoor [1,2], Richard A Hubner [1,2], Prakash Manoharan [4], Sarah O'Dwyer [2,3] and Juan W Valle [1,2,*]

1. Medical Oncology Department, The Christie NHS Foundation Trust, Manchester M20 4BX, UK; Jorge.Barriuso@manchester.ac.uk (J.B.); mairead.mcnamara@christie.nhs.uk (M.G.M.); Melissa.Frizziero@christie.nhs.uk (M.F.); Was.Mansoor@christie.nhs.uk (W.M.); Richard.Hubner@christie.nhs.uk (R.A.H.)
2. Division of Cancer Sciences, University of Manchester, Manchester M13 9PL, UK; Sarah.O'Dwyer@christie.nhs.uk
3. Surgery Department, Colorectal and Peritoneal Oncology Centre, The Christe NHS Foundation Trust, Manchester M20 4BX, UK; Hamish.Clouston@christie.nhs.uk
4. Radiology and Nuclear Medicine Department, The Christie NHS Foundation Trust, Manchester M20 4BX, UK; Prakash.Manoharan@christie.nhs.uk
* Correspondence: angela.lamarca@christie.nhs.uk (A.L.); juan.valle@christie.nhs.uk (J.W.V.)

Received: 23 August 2019; Accepted: 27 September 2019; Published: 5 October 2019

Abstract: The incidence of neuroendocrine neoplasms (NENs) is increasing, especially for patients with early stages and grade 1 tumours. Current evidence also shows increased prevalence, probably reflecting earlier stage diagnosis and improvement of treatment options. Definition of adequate postsurgical follow-up for NENs is a current challenge. There are limited guidelines, and heterogeneity in adherence to those available is notable. Unfortunately, the population of patients at greatest risk of recurrence has not been defined clearly. Some studies support that for patients with pancreatic neuroendocrine tumours (PanNETs), factors such as primary tumour (T), stage, grade (Ki-67), tumour size, and lymph node metastases (N) are of relevance. For bronchial neuroendocrine tumours (LungNETs) and small intestinal neuroendocrine tumours (siNETs), similar factors have been identified. This review summarises the evidence supporting the rationale behind follow-up after curative resection in well-differentiated PanNETs, siNETs, and LungNETS. Published evidence informing relapse rate, disease-free survival, and relapse patterns are discussed, together with an overview of current guidelines informing postsurgical investigations and duration of follow-up.

Keywords: neuroendocrine tumours; neuroendocrine neoplasms; curative surgery; resection; follow-up; guidelines; relapse; recurrence; risk factor

1. Introduction

Neuroendocrine neoplasms (NENs) are rare and heterogeneous [1,2]. Assessment of stage, primary tumour site, and tumour grade are the cornerstones for treatment planning [3,4].

For gastro-entero-pancreatic (GEP)-NENs, the World Health Organisation (WHO) tumour grade is defined by the percentage of tumour cells with a nuclear expression of Ki-67 and morphological differentiation features (well-differentiated (called neuroendocrine tumour (NET)) vs. poorly-differentiated (called neuroendocrine carcinoma (NEC))) [5–7]. Following these criteria,

GEP-NENs are classified as follows: grade (G) 1-NET (Ki-67 < 3%; well-differentiated morphology), G2-NET (Ki-67 3–20%; well-differentiated morphology), G3-NET (Ki-67 > 20%; well-differentiated morphology), and G3-NEC (Ki-67 > 20%; poorly-differentiated morphology). Lung-NENs are divided according to morphology into lung carcinoids (well-differentiated morphology) and lung NECs (poorly-differentiated morphology). Lung carcinoids are subdivided into Typical Lung Carcinoid (defined as <2 mitosis per 10 high-power fields (HPF) and absence of necrosis) and Atypical Lung Carcinoid (defined as 2–10 mitosis per 10 HPF and focal necrosis). Lung NECs are characterised by >10 mitosis per 10 HPF and diffuse necrosis and can be subdivided into large and small cell lung NECs according to cell morphology [8,9]. The role of Ki-67 in lung NETs has not been validated [10].

For patients with localised disease, surgery is the treatment of choice, especially for G1 and G2 NETs [11–13]. There is no clear evidence supporting adjuvant treatment for resected NETs [11,13], and scarce retrospective evidence available, mainly focused on lung NECs and high risk PanNETs [14,15]. Advanced disease is only amenable to palliative treatment with the aim of prolonging overall survival [13,16].

While multiple clinical trials have explored the most suitable treatment strategies for patients with advanced disease [16], the optimal postsurgical follow-up for patients with resected NENs remains unclear, with no prospective clinical trials in this setting, and variable adherence to current guidelines [17]. The definition of adequate post-resection follow-up for NENs is one of the challenges currently faced by both individual clinicians and multidisciplinary teams.

This review summarises the available evidence supporting follow-up after curative resection of sporadic (nonhereditary) well-differentiated NETs arising from the pancreas (PanNETs), small intestine (excluding appendix) (siNETs), and lung (LungNETS). This manuscript also reviews current guidelines and identifies areas of uncertainty to be addressed by future research. Since surgery for poorly-differentiated tumours has a limited role, the focus of these recommendations will be limited to patients with well-differentiated tumours. In addition, this manuscript will not cover specific recommendations for NETs arising from the appendix or rectum.

2. How Large Is the "Resected" Population?

Both the incidence and prevalence of patients with localised NETs is gradually increasing, and consequently [1], the amount of patients with resected NETs who would meet criteria for postsurgical follow-up is also increasing. There is therefore a clear need to define the best follow-up following resection. The latest evidence from the Surveillance, Epidemiology, and End Results (SEER) programme analysed 64,971 cases of NENs, and confirmed an increase in incidence with an age-adjusted annual incidence rate increase by 6.4-fold from 1973 (1.09 per 100,000) to 2012 (6.98 per 100,000) [1]. This increase occurred across all sites, stages, and grades. The highest incidences were recorded for Lung NENs (1.49 per 100,000), followed by GEP NENs (3.56 per 100,000), and NENs from an unknown primary (0.84 per 100,000). In addition, the highest incidence increase was recorded for localised stage disease (from 0.21 per 100,000 persons in 1973 to 3.15 per 100,000 persons in 2012; p value < 0.001) and G1-NETs (increased from 0.01 per 100,000 persons in 1973 to 2.53 per 100,000 persons in 2012; p value < 0.001) [1]. Whether this is a true incidence increase or an improved recognition and diagnosis remains unclear.

The median overall survival (OS) for all NENs (regardless of primary site, stage at diagnosis, or grade) was 9.3 years. As expected, longer OS (median >30 years) was reported for patients with localised (resectable) NENs when compared to those with regional (locally advanced) (median OS 10.2 years) and distant (metastatic) NENs (median OS 12 months) (p value < 0.001) [1]. Taking into account that 52.3% (28,031 out of 53,565) of the population presented with localised disease, and the prolonged OS in this population, the 20 year limited-duration prevalence also increased, from 0.006% in 1993 to 0.048% in 2012 (p value < 0.001).

3. There Is a Need to Standardise Current Practice

Even though guidelines for the postsurgical resection of PanNETs, siNETs, and LungNETS [11,18–21] are available, a recent study by Chan et al. showed that these are far from being widely adopted by clinicians, and that practice is heterogeneous [17]. Published in 2018, this practice survey of the Commonwealth Neuroendocrine Tumour Collaboration (CommNETS) and the North American Neuroendocrine Tumor Society (NANETS) gathered information regarding follow-up patterns by health care practitioners and identified areas of variation in practice [17]. A total of 163 responses to a web-based survey targeting NET health care providers in Australia, New Zealand, Canada, and the United States were received. Responding specialties included 50% medical oncology, 23% surgery, and 13% nuclear medicine (with 15% other). A large proportion of responders confirmed they were aware of follow-up guidelines, such as those from the National Comprehensive Cancer Network (NCCN) (38%), the European Neuroendocrine Tumor Society (ENETS)) (33%), and the European Society for Medical Oncology (ESMO) (17%). In contrast, only 15%, 27%, and 10%, respectively, found these guidelines "very useful", and 63% reported not to use them. Responders agreed that grade, followed by Ki-67, was the most relevant prognostic factor in the population of patients with resected NENs, while the site of origin was not felt to be of much relevance. Around half of responders reported that they followed-up resected patients for longer than 5 years (26% 6–10 years; 23% >10 years). The frequency at which such follow-up was performed varied across responders (the majority performed 3–6 monthly visits during the first 1–2 years, followed by annual visits thereafter), as did the investigations carried out at follow-up (serum tumour markers (Chromogranin A (CgA) 86%) and computerised tomography (CT 66%) were the more frequently employed tests). Only 40% of responders performed radiological assessment after the first 5 years of follow-up post-resection [17]. No other studies exploring this issue are available to date.

These results highlight the huge variability in practice and in adherence to current guidelines. One of the reasons for such poor adoption may be the lack of high quality evidence behind the available recommendations, together with the lack of evidence to favour specific follow-up tools over others. This variability in follow-up can explain not only the lack of quality retrospective data (unreliable in view of different follow-up strategies adopted across countries/centres), but also the challenges in identifying populations at increased risk of relapse, which may enable prospective development of adjuvant strategies.

It is therefore of major importance to work towards an improved standardisation of follow-up for patients with resected NETs.

4. Why? Rationale for Follow-Up

Current guidelines are available with post curative resection follow-up recommendations for all patients diagnosed with PanNETs [11,18,19,22,23], siNETs [18,21–23], and LungNETs [11,18,22,23].

The main factor supporting long-term postsurgical follow-up is not only the risk of recurrence, but the risk of late recurrence. The duration of post curative resection follow-up seems to be associated with the risk of later recurrence and recommendations are individualised for each cancer subtype. The risk of breast cancer recurrence continues through 15 years after primary treatment and beyond, and based on this, long-term mammography is recommended [24]. In contrast, for lung and colorectal cancer, most recurrences will occur within the first 2 years (maximum of 5 years) from the time of curative surgery, and current guidelines recommend follow-up for up to 5 years after curative resection [25,26].

It is anticipated that through regular follow-up, relapse should be diagnosed earlier, when surgical strategies with curative intent may be of benefit [27]. Benefits of postsurgical follow-up have shown to translate into significant improvements in patient overall survival in patients with breast cancer [28]. Evidence in colorectal cancer varies between studies, with some studies suggesting a benefit in terms of overall survival [26], while others showed a minimal impact on survival benefit despite higher rate

4.1. Resected PanNETs

Multiple retrospective series have explored the risk of relapse following surgery for PanNETs. Some of the most recent series are summarised in Table 1 [30–34]. Risk of tumour recurrence varied between series (12%–25%–69%) [30,34,35], as did the reported disease-free survival (19–55 months) [30,33]. In the series published by Sho and colleagues, patients diagnosed with PanNETs who underwent surgical resection between 1989 and 2015 were reported [31]. Of the 140 patients included, relapse-free survival dropped significantly after 5 years of follow-up (5 and 10 year relapse-free survival was 84.6% and 67.1%, respectively). It is also worth noting that some series have reported shorter disease-free survivals for PanNETs (vs. other NETs). In a series reporting data of over 900 patients with NETs, the median DFS among patients with resected siNET or PanNETs was 5.8 and 4.1 years, respectively [36]. Similar trends were reported by Singh et al. [35]. Such findings, together with identification of tumour recurrence after 10 years of follow-up [34,35], suggest that long-term follow-up is required for PanNETs. Some of the series did highlight an incongruence between the pattern of follow-up imaging performed (more frequent assessment during the first 3 years postsurgery) and the time-to-recurrence reported (only one third of patients recurred over this period of time. Cumulative incidence of recurrence was 26.5%, 39.6%, 57.0%, and 69.4% at 3, 5, 10, and 15 years post-resection, respectively [35].

The site of tumour recurrence has been described to be predominantly distant, with a tropism for liver metastases [31,34,37]. Rates of local recurrence are variable between series [32]. There seems to be an increased rate of pancreas-only recurrence associated with surgical margin status [38].

Table 1. Most relevant retrospective series in PanNETs.

Author; Year	Relapse Rate	Risk Factors	Site of Recurrence
Gao et al. 2018 [30]	Relapse rate 129/505 (25.5%). Median disease-free survival of 19 months (range 6–96 months).	T3, T4, N+, Ki-67 >2%, functional	Not reported
Sho et al. 2018 [31]	Relapse rate 23/140 (16.3%). 5 and 10 year relapse-free survival was 84.6% and 67.1%, respectively.	Size >5 cm, N+, Ki-67 >20%	All recurrence was distant (liver, peritoneal, and bone)
Genç et al. 2018 [32]	Relapse rate 35/211 (17%). The 5 and 10 year disease-specific/overall survival was 98%/91% and 84%/68%, respectively. Median time to recurrence was 43 months (IQR 23–62).	Grade 2, N+, perineural invasion	Pancreatic remnant (69%), distant (14%), 1 patients had lymph node metastasis
Ausania et al. 2019 [33]	Relapse rate 19/137 (13.9%). Median DFS was 55 months.	Tumour size >2 cm, N+, Ki-67>5% or mitotic index >2	Not reported
Marchegiani et al. 2018 [34]	Relapse rate (12.3%) Recurrence occurred either during the first year of follow-up ($n = 9$), or after ten years ($n = 4$).	>21 mm size, G3, N+, vascular infiltration	Liver (11.1%), local recurrence (2.3%), lymph node (2.1%), other organs (1.6%)
Singh et al. 2018 [35]	Cumulative incidence of recurrence was 26.5%, 39.6%, 57.0%, 69.4% at 3, 5, 10 and 15 years post-resection, respectively.	Not reported	Not reported

Summary of the latest and largest retrospective series exploring relapse rate and risk of relapse for patients diagnosed with resected pancreatic neuroendocrine tumours (PanNETs) [30–35]. n, number; N, lymph node; N+, affected lymph node; T, primary tumour; IQR, interquartile range; DFS, disease-free survival; G, grade.

4.2. Resected siNETs

Despite expected indolent clinical behaviour, the risk of relapse reported seems to vary according to the length of follow-up between studies [35,36]. In a series of 936 patients (of whom 43 were siNETs), the cumulative incidence of recurrence for the siNET population was 22.8%, 33.8%, 52.9%, and 62.0% at 3, 5, 10 and 15 years post-resection, respectively [35]. In view of the risk of relapse even a long time after resection, long-term follow-up is recommended. As previously mentioned, disease-free survival seems to be longer for siNETs than for PanNETs, with median disease-free survivals varying among studies [35,36].

The relapse sites have been reported to be distant, with liver predominance [36].

4.3. Resected LungNETs

Some retrospective series have explored the risk of recurrence following resection of LungNETs. The series by Lou and colleagues reported a 6% recurrence rate after a median follow-up time of 3.5 years within a population of 337 patients with resected LungNETs. Sites of recurrence were mainly distant, with predominance of liver and bone metastases [39]. Of the 21 patients with tumour recurrence, only one had evidence of local relapse. Whether longer time of follow-up would impact the relapse rate reported remains unclear. Current guidelines recommend long-term follow-up in view of risk of late relapse (up to 19% of relapses were 7 years from resection in some series) reported in the literature [40,41].

5. For Whom? Risk Stratification

As specified above, and in view of the risk of tumour recurrence, current guidelines recommend follow-up for all resected patients with PanNETs, siNETs, and LungNETs [11,18–21]. However, recommendations from current guidelines provide few insights regarding individualised recommendations based on individual tumour characteristics, which may derive an increased relapse risk. Thus, risk stratification may be of relevance not only to reduce exposure to radiation in these patients with lower risk, but also to ensure adequate use of resources and to identify target populations for future clinical trials in the adjuvant setting. Some recent publications provide initial recommendations that tailor the frequency of follow-up investigations to tumour characteristics such as size, Ki-67, or lymph node metastases, but these are not yet adopted by international guidelines [42–44]. Development of molecular markers for risk of recurrence stratification are under development, but remain investigational and not available for its use in daily clinical practice [45].

5.1. Resected PanNETs

Reported series are consistent regarding the increased risk of relapse related to tumour size (>2 cm), presence of lymph node metastases in the resection specimen (N+), grade 2 tumours (vs. grade 1), and the presence of involved microscopic resection margins (R1) (vs. clear resection margins (R0)) [30–34,44]. Other factors such as Ki-67 above 5%, tumour functionality, and the presence of perineural and vascular invasion have also been suggested as factors related to increased relapse risk. However, these observations are not consistent between series and are likely to require further validation [30,32,34,46]. It is considered that resected insulinomas with N0 and R0 disease are the PanNETs with the lowest risk of tumour recurrence [19]. There has been recent evidence supporting the impact not only of presence/absence of affected lymph nodes, but also the number of these. Partelli and colleagues showed that the presence of 4 or more lymph node metastases (N2 disease) correlated with a lower 3 year disease-free survival (75%) when compared with presence of 1-3 positive lymph nodes (N1 disease; 3 year disease free survival rate of 83%) and N0 disease (3 year disease free survival rate of 89%) [47]. Authors also suggested that a minimum of 13 examined lymph nodes seemed to be adequate for such assessment [47].

5.2. Resected siNETs

One of the most relevant risk factors to predict increased relapse risk in patients with siNETs is the presence of lymph node metastases in the resected specimen. Zaidi and colleagues reported a series of 199 patients with resected siNETs [48]. Of the whole population, 154 patients (77.4%) had lymph node-positive disease. No difference in 3 year recurrence-free survival was found between patients with lymph node-positive (N+) and lymph node-negative (N0) disease. However, authors demonstrated that patients with four or more positive lymph nodes had a worse 3 year recurrence-free survival (81.6% vs. 1–3 (91.4%) or 0 (92.1%) lymph nodes affected; p value 0.01). In addition, the authors also concluded that retrieval of eight or more lymph nodes at time of surgery was required to accurately evaluate number of lymph nodes involved. Other risk factors such as grade (grade 2; especially if Ki-67 > 10%) and T3/4 tumours have also been reported [35,36].

5.3. Resected LungNETs

Risk factors associated with increased relapse risk for LungNETs include the presence of positive lymph nodes (N+) [39,49] and the presence of atypical LungNETs (26%; vs. 3% in typical LungNETs) for whom time to recurrence was also shorter (median 1.8 years (range 0.2–7 years) vs. 4 years (range 0.8–12 years) for typical LungNETs) [39]. Other series have also reported that mitotic index, Ki-67 index, and the presence of necrosis were independent prognostic factors for relapse-free survival in resected LungNETs [10].

6. How? Presurgical Staging and Follow-Up Tools

In addition to patient history and physical examination, cross-sectional imaging (both in the form of CT and magnetic resonance imaging (MRI)) is one of the main tools for patient follow-up. Reduction of exposure to radiation is to be considered when planning for long-term follow-up, especially in young patients, and alternating CT and MRI (or limiting to MRI alone) could be an alternative in selected scenarios [50]. In addition, use of serum/urine biomarkers and nuclear medicine imaging have a role that warrants further discussion [23]. Table 2 provides a summary of the recommendations for each one of the assessments discussed in this section [11,18–23], both for baseline assessment and follow-up. Table 3 provides a summary of further recommendations, including timing and frequency of examinations suggested by current guidelines [11,18–23].

6.1. Currently-Available Biomarkers

Histologically, NETs share common features, such as specific secretory granules often containing biogenic amines and polypeptide hormones that help with the diagnostic process. Chromogranin and synaptophysin are examples of tumour markers utilised, while neuron-specific enolase (NSE) is less specific [51]. The use of staining with peptide hormones, such as insulin, glucagon, or other specific peptides is of use in selected cases only, when such diagnoses as insulinoma, glucagonoma, etc. are suspected [52].

Serum/urine markers can be useful not only for diagnosis in patients with NETs, but also for follow-up. Serum markers of relevance include Chromogranin A (CgA), which is co-secreted with other hormones by neuroendocrine tumour cells [52]. Only 10%–40% of PanNETs are functioning tumours [19]. Based on this, measurement of serum pancreatic polypeptide, insulin, glucagon, somatostatin, gastrin, vasoactive intestinal polypeptide (VIP), and others has a role if patients' symptoms suggest a particular diagnosis related to these secretions [19]. In patients with siNETs, quantification of 5-hydroxyindoleacetic acid (5-HIAA), a metabolite of serotonin, in either serum or urine is recommended [53]. The use of serum NSE is usually limited to poorly-differentiated NECs [54], with some evidence suggesting its role for atypical LungNETs [55].

In the setting of localised resectable disease, baseline assessment (preferably presurgery) of the above-mentioned serum/urine tumour markers could inform which the most suitable serum marker for follow-up after surgery on an individual patient basis is [52]. However, clinicians should bear in mind potential false positive findings when performing biochemistry follow-up [56]. Discrepancy between guidelines exists in this setting, and while most guidelines support the role of biochemistry follow-up for patients with resected NETs [11,18–21,23], the CommNETs/NANETS guidelines do not fully support such an approach outside the scenario of patients with functioning PanNETs [22].

While other novel biomarkers are currently being developed, their use has not been validated in this setting [57–59].

Table 2. Summary recommendations of baseline and follow-up tools in assessment of patients after curative resection of neuroendocrine tumours. Adapted from [11,18–21].

		Biochemistry				Cross-Sectional Imaging (CT/MRI)	SSTR Imaging (^{68}Ga-DOTA-PET)	^{18}F-FDG-PET
		CgA (Serum)	5-HIAA (Serum/Urine)	Pancreatic Peptides (Serum)	NSE			
PanNETs	First assessment	✓	×	If functional	×	✓	✓	×
	Follow-up	✓	×	If functional	×	✓	**	×
siNETs	First-assessment	✓	✓	×	×	✓	✓	×
	Follow-up	✓	If elevated at diagnosis	×	×	✓	**	×
LungNETs	First assessment	✓	✓	×	If atypical	✓	✓	If atypical
	Follow-up	✓	If elevated at diagnosis	×	If elevated at diagnosis	✓	**	#

PanNETs, well-differentiated pancreatic neuroendocrine tumours; siNETs, well-differentiated small intestinal neuroendocrine tumours; LungNETs, well-differentiated lung carcinoids (typical/atypical); CgA, chromogranin A; 5-HIAA, 5-hydroxyindoleacetic acid; NSE, neuron-specific enolase; CT, computerised tomography; MRI, magnetic resonance imaging; SSTR, somatostatin receptor; PET, positron-emission tomography; ^{18}F-FDG, fluorodeoxyglucose; ^{68}Ga-DOTA, 68Ga-dodecanetetraacetic acid. ** According to the ENETS guidelines, follow-up with SSTR imaging if positive at diagnosis could be considered. # According to the ENETS guidelines, follow-up with ^{18}F-FDG PET, if positive at diagnosis could be considered for atypical LungNETs; ✓ Recommended; × Not recommended.

Table 3. Summary of patient outcomes and follow-up recommendations. Outcome data extracted from [30–35]. Recommendations adapted from [11,18–23].

						Staging	Follow-Up Recommendations (ENETS, NCCN, CommNETs/NANETS)		
	Relapse Rate	Late Relapse	Site of Recurrence / Metastases	Risk Factors for Relapse		Pre-Surgery	3–12 Month Post-Resection	After 1st Year and Until 10 Years Post-Resection	After 10 Years
PanNETs	12%–25% up to 70% at 15 years of follow-up	>5–10 years	Liver > local	Size/T, N, Ki-67/grade		Cross-sectional imaging (CT/MRI) + SSTR imaging * (+ pancreatic peptides if functioning)	History and physical examination + biochemistry* + cross-sectional imaging (CT/MRI)	Frequency: 3–6 monthly for nonfunctional PanNETs and 6–12 monthly for functional PanNETs (ENETS) / 6–12 monthly (NCCN) / every year for 3 years, every 1–2 years thereafter (CommNETs/NANETS). As per ENETS guidelines insulinomas may not require any radiological follow-up. Examinations: History and physical examination + biochemistry* + cross-sectional imaging (CT/MRI) ENETS guidelines suggest 1–2 yearly SSTR imaging if positive at diagnosis	Individualised decision to continue; recommended life-long (ENETS)

Table 3. Cont.

	Relapse Rate	Late Relapse	Site of Recurrence / Metastases	Risk Factors for Relapse	Staging Pre-Surgery	Staging 3-12 Month Post-Resection	Follow-up Recommendations (ENETS, NCCN, CommNETs/NANETS) After 1st Year and Until 10 Years Post-Resection	Follow-up After 10 Years
siNETs	20%–50%; up to 62% at 15 years of follow-up	10–15 years	Liver	Resected number of lymph nodes (>8) and positivity of those lymph nodes (>4)	Cross-sectional imaging (CT/MRI) + SSTR imaging + CgA (+ 5-HIAA)	History and physical examination + biochemistry * + cross-sectional imaging (CT/MRI)	Frequency: 6-12 monthly (ENETS) / every 1-2 years (CommNETs/NANETS/NCCN). Examinations: History and physical examination + biochemistry * + cross-sectional imaging (CT/MRI). ENETS guidelines suggest 2 yearly SSTR imaging if positive at diagnosis	Individualised decision to continue; recommended life-long (ENETS)
LungNETs	3%–26% depending on subtype	>7 years; atypical developed earlier relapse	Liver and bone	Mitotic index, Ki-67, necrosis, atypical, N	Cross-sectional imaging (CT/MRI) + SSTR imaging [18F-FDG-PET could be considered if atypical] + CgA (+ 5-HIAA + NSE [if atypical])		Frequency: 6-12 monthly (ENETS/NCCN); 3-6 monthly if atypical (ENETS). Examinations: History and physical examination + biochemistry * + cross-sectional imaging (CT/MRI) ENETS guidelines suggest 1–3 yearly SSTR imaging if positive at diagnosis (1–2 yearly for atypical); 18F-FDG PET could be considered for atypical tumour if positive at diagnosis; ENETS guidelines also support the use of 5–10 yearly bronchoscopy for follow-up if positive at diagnosis (every 1–3 years for atypical LungNETs)	Individualised decision to continue; recommended life-long (ENETS)

PanNETs, well-differentiated pancreatic neuroendocrine tumours; siNETs, well-differentiated small intestinal neuroendocrine tumours; LungNETs, well-differentiated lung carcinoids (typical/atypical); N, lymph node; T, primary tumour; CT, computerised tomography; MRI, magnetic resonance imaging; CgA, chromogranin A; SSTR, somatostatin receptor; 5-HIAA, 5-hydroxyindoleacetic acid; NSE, neuron-specific enolase; 18F-FDG, fluorodeoxyglucose; PET, positron-emission tomography. * not fully supported by the CommNETs/NANETS guidelines [22] with the exception of functional PanNET.

6.2. The Evolving Role of Nuclear Medicine

One of the suggested reasons for the increasing incidence of NETs is the improvement in diagnostic imaging techniques [60]. ^{18}Fluoro-deoxyglucose (^{18}F-FDG), was one of the first tracers developed in oncology. However, its role in the diagnosis and/or follow-up of NENs is considered more relevant in patients with poorly-differentiated NENs [13,61–65].

The expression of somatostatin receptors (SSTR) on the cell membrane is one of the unique characteristics of NETs, which makes SSTRs a suitable molecular target for specific diagnostic and therapeutic ligands. Based on this, the nuclear medicine field has targeted SSTRs for diagnosis and treatment of NETs for decades [66]. The vast majority of research has been focused on Indium-111 (^{111}In)-pentetreotide (Octreoscan®), which was the only approved agent for the scintigraphic localisation of primary and metastatic NETs [67]. More recently, the clinical use of gallium-68 (^{68}Ga)-labelled compounds has increased in NETs [68,69] due to its affinity for multiple SSTR subtypes (SSTR2, SSTR3, SSTR5) [70]. In addition, the first Ready-to-Use (SOMAKIT TOC®) ^{68}Ga-DOTA0-Tyr3-Octreotide (^{68}Ga-DOTATOC) for injection was approved for use in patients diagnosed with GEP-NETs [71].

In the last decade, several clinical studies have compared the diagnostic role of ^{68}Ga-DOTA-PET to somatostatin receptor scintigraphy (Octreoscan®) in patients diagnosed with NETs. These studies have confirmed an increased sensitivity and image quality, together with an increased capacity to detect additional lesions and alter management in favour of ^{68}Ga-DOTA-PET [72–78].

A recent systematic review and meta-analysis of 22 studies exploring the role of ^{68}Ga-DOTA-PET in NETs reported a high pooled sensitivity (93% (95% CI 91%–94%)) and specificity (96% (95% CI 95%–98%)) [79]. The only exceptions to this high performance are insulinomas, for which lower sensitivities have been reported [80]. In addition, the use of ^{68}Ga-DOTA-PET in PanNETs has been reported to provide useful additional information, and impacted on patient management, in 20%–55% of cases [81–84].

For LungNETs, studies have reported a more selective uptake of ^{68}Ga-DOTA for typical LungNETs, while atypical LungNETs demonstrated less ^{68}Ga-DOTA uptake and increased ^{18}F-FDG avidity [85].

A retrospective series of 46 patients with LungNETs assessed with ^{68}Ga-DOTA-PET reported that the ^{68}Ga-DOTA-PET provided additional information in 37% of patients and impacted on management in 26% [78]. A change in management was due to identification of occult sites in nine patients, three of whom were patients in the postsurgical setting. No differences in the rate of practice-changing ^{68}Ga-DOTA-PET results by type of LungNET were reported in this series.

Based on the above evidence, SSTR imaging (preferably in the form of ^{68}Ga-DOTA-PET, if available) is the method of choice to fully stage patients with PanNETs, siNETs and LungNETs [19,21]. Such examination is recommended as a baseline assessment (preferably presurgery) or as a baseline postoperative assessment only (preferably after 3–6 months from surgery to avoid false positive findings [86]). Current guidelines do not recommend the use of nuclear medicine imaging for routine surveillance [11,18–21], with the exception of the ENETS guidelines which suggest consideration of SSTR imaging 2 yearly following resection for patients with known positive SSTRs before surgery [23]. Once again, possibility of false positive findings may challenge interpretation of results and should be taken into account by treating clinicians [87].

7. Summary of Current Guidelines

Current guidelines recommend post curative resection follow-up for all patients diagnosed with PanNETs [11,18,19,22,23], siNETs [18,21–23], and LungNETs [11,18,22,23]. Table 3 provides a summary of recommendations from current ENETS, NCCN, and CommNETs/NANETS guidelines [11,18–23]. Recommendations regarding who the most appropriate specialist is to perform such follow up do not exist.

Even though most guidelines available agree regarding the type of investigations to be performed, the frequency of such examinations varies significantly between them. In addition, follow-up beyond 10 years is suggested as a discussion point to have with patients on an individual patient basis by the

NCCN and CommNETs/NANETS guidelines, while the ENETS guidelines suggest life-long follow-up for well-differentiated NETs. Finally, biochemistry follow-up is not strongly recommended by the CommNETs/NANETS guidelines, in view of the limited impact on patient management, with the exception of functional PanNETs [22]. ENETS guidelines also suggest the role of regular postsurgical SSTR imaging in patients with known previous uptake pre-resection [23].

8. Conclusions and Future Steps

The available literature confirms that following resection of well-differentiated NETs, and despite their "indolent" behaviour, relapse rate can be frequent, especially if long-term follow-up is adopted [35]. Reported relapse rates vary between series, probably due to the variability regarding follow-up recommendations between available guidelines, together with lack of adherence to such guidelines, not only between countries but also between centres in the same country [17]. Some of the main discrepancies between the available guidelines are related to the frequency of assessments, the role of biochemistry follow-up, and the role of SSTR imaging. Unless prospective studies are pursued to clarify the real benefit and impact of such investigations on patients' outcome, these will remain unclear with continued practice variability. The risk/benefit ratio of degree of exposure to radiation does also require to be taken into account. The development of novel biomarkers should be exposed to scrutiny with mandated validation before being adopted into guidelines.

In view of the increasing incidence of NETs, mainly in the form of localised stages, standardisation of follow-up strategies with the potential to increase cure rate is becoming an urgent need for the field to move forward. In order to achieve such an impact, development of adjuvant strategies in NETs will need to be explored. Few studies have explored this and there are many associated challenges. Firstly, NETs are rare tumours, and when focusing on a resectable patient population potentially eligible for clinical trials, recruitment may be a barrier, unless studies are designed within international networks. Secondly, the heterogeneity of NETs would make it mandatory for trials to focus on specific patient populations (PanNETs, siNETs, or LungNETs) which would be an additional challenge to recruitment. Thirdly, and in view of long-term relapse patterns, such clinical trials would require long-term follow-up with the associated cost. A potential solution for this would be to focus on patients with an increased risk of tumour recurrence, allowing for stratification based on the available retrospective evidence. Finally, based on the high rate of distant relapse, systemic treatment would need to be explored, if an adjuvant study was to be designed.

In summary, current guidelines and clinical practice vary regarding follow-up recommendations in patients with NETs. Standardised practice and agreement between guidelines is required to secure homogeneity of follow-up, better identification of patients at risk of recurrence, and an adequate study design exploring adjuvant strategies in patients with NETs to increase the cure rate statistics. Prospective studies performed in this setting, together with high quality patient registries, are required to move the field forward.

Author Contributions: A.L. drafted the manuscript; All authors: approved the final version of the manuscript.

Funding: A.L. received funding from The Christie Charity. J.B. received funding from the ENETS Centre of Excellence Fellowship Grant Award. M.F. received an ENETS Centre of Excellence Young Investigator Grant 2018.

Conflicts of Interest: Authors have no conflicts of interest to declare related to this manuscript.

References

1. Dasari, A.; Shen, C.; Halperin, D.; Zhao, B.; Zhou, S.; Xu, Y.; Shih, T.; Yao, J.C. Trends in the Incidence, Prevalence, and Survival Outcomes in Patients With Neuroendocrine Tumors in the United States. *JAMA Oncol.* **2017**, *3*, 1335–1342. [CrossRef] [PubMed]
2. Auernhammer, C.J.; Spitzweg, C.; Angele, M.K.; Boeck, S. Advanced neuroendocrine tumours of the small intestine and pancreas: Clinical developments, controversies, and future strategies. *Lancet Diabetes Endocrinol.* **2017**, *6*, 404–415. [CrossRef]

3. Lloyd, R.V.; Osamura, R.Y.; Kloppel, G.; Rosai, J. *WHO Classification of Tumours: Pathology and Genetics of Tumours of Endocrine Organs*; IARC: Lyon, France, 2017.
4. Bosman, F.T.; Carneiro, F.; Hruban, R.H.; Theise, N.D. *WHO Classification of Tumours of the Digestive System*; World Health Organization: Geneva, Switzerland, 2010.
5. Rindi, G.; Klersy, C.; Inzani, F.; Fellegara, G. Grading the neuroendocrine tumors of the lung: An evidence-based proposal. *Endocr. Relat. Cancer* **2014**, *21*, 1–16. [CrossRef]
6. Rindi, G.; Arnold, R.; Bosman, F.T.; Capella, C.; Klimstra, D.S.; Klöppel, G.; Komminoth, P.; Solcia, E. Nomenclature and classification of neuroendocrine neoplasms of the digestive system. In *WHO Classification of Tumours of the Digestive System*, 4th ed.; Bosman, T.F., Carneiro, F., Hruban, R.H., Theise, N.D., Eds.; International Agency for Research on cancer (IARC): Lyon, France, 2010; p. 13.
7. Klöppel, G.C.A.; Hruban, R.H. Neoplasms of the neuroendocrine pancreas. In *WHO Classification of Tumours of the Endocrine Organs*; IARC Press: Lyon, France, 2017; pp. 210–239.
8. Travis WDBEM-HHKH. The concept of pulmonary neuroendocrine tumours. In *Pathology & Genetics: Tumours of the Lung, Pleura, Thymus, and Heart*; IARC Press: Lyon, France, 2004; p. 19.
9. Pelosi, G.; Fabbri, A.; Cossa, M.; Sonzogni, A.; Valeri, B.; Righi, L.; Papotti, M. What clinicians are asking pathologists when dealing with lung neuroendocrine neoplasms? *Semin. Diagn. Pathol.* **2015**, *32*, 469–479. [CrossRef] [PubMed]
10. Clay, V.; Papaxoinis, G.; Sanderson, B.; Valle, J.W.; Howell, M.; Lamarca, A.; Krysiak, P.; Bishop, P.; Nonaka, D.; Mansoor, W. Evaluation of diagnostic and prognostic significance of Ki-67 index in pulmonary carcinoid tumours. *Clin. Transl. Oncol.* **2017**, *19*, 579–586. [CrossRef] [PubMed]
11. Caplin, M.E.; Baudin, E.; Ferolla, P.; Filosso, P.; Garcia-Yuste, M.; Lim, E.; Oberg, K.; Pelosi, G.; Perren, A.; Rossi, R.E.; et al. Pulmonary neuroendocrine (carcinoid) tumors: European Neuroendocrine Tumor Society expert consensus and recommendations for best practice for typical and atypical pulmonary carcinoids. *Ann. Oncol.* **2015**, *26*, 1604–1620. [CrossRef] [PubMed]
12. Delle Fave, G.; O'Toole, D.; Sundin, A.; Taal, B.; Ferolla, P.; Ramage, J.K.; Ferone, D.; Ito, T.; Weber, W.; Zheng-Pei, Z.; et al. ENETS Consensus Guidelines Update for Gastroduodenal Neuroendocrine Neoplasms. *Neuroendocrinology* **2016**, *103*, 119–124. [CrossRef] [PubMed]
13. Garcia-Carbonero, R.; Sorbye, H.; Baudin, E.; Raymond, E.; Wiedenmann, B.; Niederle, B.; Sedlackova, E.; Toumpanakis, C.; Anlauf, M.; Cwikla, J.B.; et al. ENETS Consensus Guidelines for High-Grade Gastroenteropancreatic Neuroendocrine Tumors and Neuroendocrine Carcinomas. *Neuroendocrinology* **2016**, *103*, 186–194. [CrossRef] [PubMed]
14. Raman, V.; Jawitz, O.K.; Yang, C.J.; Tong, B.C.; D'Amico, T.A.; Berry, M.F.; Harpole, D.H., Jr. Adjuvant Therapy for Patients With Early Large Cell Lung Neuroendocrine Cancer: A National Analysis. *Ann. Thorac. Surg.* **2019**, *108*, 377–383. [CrossRef] [PubMed]
15. Arvold, N.D.; Willett, C.G.; Fernandez-del Castillo, C.; Ryan, D.P.; Ferrone, C.R.; Clark, J.W.; Blaszkowsky, L.S.; Deshpande, V.; Niemierko, A.; Allen, J.N.; et al. Pancreatic neuroendocrine tumors with involved surgical margins: Prognostic factors and the role of adjuvant radiotherapy. *Int. J. Radiat. Oncol. Biol. Phys.* **2012**, *83*, e337–e343. [CrossRef] [PubMed]
16. Pavel, M.; Valle, J.W.; Eriksson, B.; Fazio, N.; Caplin, M.; Gorbounova, V.; OConnor, J.; Eriksson, B.; Sorbye, H.; Kulke, M.; et al. ENETS Consensus Guidelines for the Standards of Care in Neuroendocrine Neoplasms: Systemic Therapy—Biotherapy and Novel Targeted Agents. *Neuroendocrinology* **2017**, *105*, 266–280. [CrossRef] [PubMed]
17. Chan, D.L.; Moody, L.; Segelov, E.; Metz, D.C.; Strosberg, J.R.; Pavlakis, N.; Singh, S. Follow-Up for Resected Gastroenteropancreatic Neuroendocrine Tumours: A Practice Survey of the Commonwealth Neuroendocrine Tumour Collaboration (CommNETS) and the North American Neuroendocrine Tumor Society (NANETS). *Neuroendocrinology* **2018**, *107*, 32–41. [CrossRef] [PubMed]
18. Sha, G. NCCN Guidelines Insights: Neuroendocrine and Adrenal Tumors, Version 2. *J. Natl. Compr. Canc. Netw.* 2018. Available online: http://oncolife.com.ua/doc/nccn/Neuroendocrine_Tumors.pdf (accessed on 27 September 2019). [CrossRef]
19. Falconi, M.; Eriksson, B.; Kaltsas, G.; Bartsch, D.K.; Capdevila, J.; Caplin, M.; Kos-Kudla, B.; Kwekkeboom, D.; Rindi, G.; Klöppel, G.; et al. ENETS Consensus Guidelines Update for the Management of Patients with Functional Pancreatic Neuroendocrine Tumors and Non-Functional Pancreatic Neuroendocrine Tumors. *Neuroendocrinology* **2016**, *103*, 153–171. [CrossRef] [PubMed]

20. Partelli, S.; Bartsch, D.K.; Capdevila, J.; Chen, J.; Knigge, U.; Niederle, B.; Nieveen van Dijkum, E.J.M.; Pape, U.F.; Pascher, A.; Ramage, J.; et al. ENETS Consensus Guidelines for Standard of Care in Neuroendocrine Tumours: Surgery for Small Intestinal and Pancreatic Neuroendocrine Tumours. *Neuroendocrinology* **2017**, *105*, 255–265. [CrossRef] [PubMed]
21. Niederle, B.; Pape, U.F.; Costa, F.; Gross, D.; Kelestimur, F.; Knigge, U.; Öberg, K.; Pavel, M.; Perren, A.; Toumpanakis, C.; et al. ENETS Consensus Guidelines Update for Neuroendocrine Neoplasms of the Jejunum and Ileum. *Neuroendocrinology* **2016**, *103*, 125–138. [CrossRef] [PubMed]
22. Singh, S.; Moody, L.; Chan, D.L.; Metz, D.C.; Strosberg, J.; Asmis, T.; Bailey, D.L.; Bergsland, E.; Brendtro, K.; Carroll, R.; et al. Follow-up Recommendations for Completely Resected Gastroenteropancreatic Neuroendocrine Tumors. *JAMA Oncol.* **2018**, *4*, 1597–1604. [CrossRef] [PubMed]
23. Knigge, U.; Capdevila, J.; Bartsch, D.K.; Baudin, E.; Falkerby, J.; Kianmanesh, R.; Kos-Kudla, B.; Niederle, B.; Nieveen van Dijkum, E.; O'Toole, D.; et al. ENETS Consensus Recommendations for the Standards of Care in Neuroendocrine Neoplasms: Follow-Up and Documentation. *Neuroendocrinology* **2017**, *105*, 310–319. [CrossRef] [PubMed]
24. Khatcheressian, J.L.; Hurley, P.; Bantug, E.; Esserman, L.J.; Grunfeld, E.; Halberg, F.; Hantel, A.; Henry, N.L.; Muss, H.B.; Smith, T.J.; et al. Breast cancer follow-up and management after primary treatment: American Society of Clinical Oncology clinical practice guideline update. *J. Clin. Oncol.* **2013**, *31*, 961–965. [CrossRef] [PubMed]
25. Aslam, R.; Biswas, A.; Blaxill, P. P74 Follow-up Of Lung Cancer Patients Post Surgery. *Thorax* **2014**, *69*, A108. [CrossRef]
26. Godhi, S.; Godhi, A.; Bhat, R.; Saluja, S. Colorectal Cancer: Postoperative Follow-up and Surveillance. *Indian J. Surg.* **2017**, *79*, 234–237. [CrossRef]
27. Frilling, A.; Modlin, I.M.; Kidd, M.; Russell, C.; Breitenstein, S.; Salem, R.; Kwekkeboom, D.; Lau, W.Y.; Klersy, C.; Vilgrain, V.; et al. Recommendations for management of patients with neuroendocrine liver metastases. *Lancet Oncol.* **2014**, *15*, e8–e21. [CrossRef]
28. Lee, J.Y.; Lim, S.H.; Lee, M.Y.; Kim, H.; Kim, M.; Kim, S.; Jung, H.A.; Sohn, I.; Gil, W.H.; Lee, J.E.; et al. Impact on Survival of Regular Postoperative Surveillance for Patients with Early Breast Cancer. *Cancer Res. Treat.* **2015**, *47*, 765–773. [CrossRef] [PubMed]
29. Primrose, J.N.; Perera, R.; Gray, A.; Rose, P.; Fuller, A.; Corkhill, A.; George, S.; Mant, D.; FACS Trial Investigators. Effect of 3 to 5 years of scheduled CEA and CT follow-up to detect recurrence of colorectal cancer: The FACS randomized clinical trial. *JAMA* **2014**, *311*, 263–270. [CrossRef] [PubMed]
30. Gao, H.; Liu, L.; Wang, W.Q.; Xu, H.M.; Jin, K.Z.; Wu, C.T.; Qi, Z.H.; Zhang, S.R.; Liu, C.; Xu, J.Z.; et al. Novel recurrence risk stratification of resected pancreatic neuroendocrine tumor. *Cancer Lett.* **2018**, *412*, 188–193. [CrossRef] [PubMed]
31. Sho, S.; Court, C.M.; Winograd, P.; Toste, P.A.; Pisegna, J.R.; Lewis, M.; Donahue, T.R.; Hines, O.J.; Reber, H.A.; Dawson, D.W.; et al. A Prognostic Scoring System for the Prediction of Metastatic Recurrence Following Curative Resection of Pancreatic Neuroendocrine Tumors. *J. Gastrointest. Surg.* **2018**, *23*, 1392–1400. [CrossRef] [PubMed]
32. Genc, C.G.; Jilesen, A.P.; Partelli, S.; Falconi, M.; Muffatti, F.; van Kemenade, F.J.; van Eeden, S.; Verheij, J.; van Dieren, S.; van Eijck, C.H.J.; et al. A New Scoring System to Predict Recurrent Disease in Grade 1 and 2 Nonfunctional Pancreatic Neuroendocrine Tumors. *Ann. Surg.* **2018**, *267*, 1148–1154. [CrossRef] [PubMed]
33. Ausania, F.; Senra Del Rio, P.; Gomez-Bravo, M.A.; Martin-Perez, E.; Pérez-Daga, J.A.; Dorcaratto, D.; González-Nicolás, T.; Sanchez-Cabus, S.; Tardio-Baiges, A.; et al. Can we predict recurrence in WHO G1-G2 pancreatic neuroendocrine neoplasms? Results from a multi-institutional Spanish study. *Pancreatology* **2019**, *19*, 367–371. [CrossRef] [PubMed]
34. Marchegiani, G.; Landoni, L.; Andrianello, S.; Masini, G.; Cingarlini, S.; D'Onofrio, M.; De Robertis, R.; Davì, M.; Capelli, P.; Manfrin, E.; et al. Patterns of Recurrence after Resection for Pancreatic Neuroendocrine Tumors: Who, When, and Where? *Neuroendocrinology* **2019**, *108*, 161–171. [CrossRef]
35. Singh, S.; Chan, D.L.; Moody, L.; Liu, N.; Fischer, H.D.; Austin, P.C.; Segelov, E. Recurrence in Resected Gastroenteropancreatic Neuroendocrine Tumors. *JAMA Oncol.* **2018**, *4*, 583–585. [CrossRef]

36. Ter-Minassian, M.; Chan, J.A.; Hooshmand, S.M.; Brais, L.K.; Daskalova, A.; Heafield, R.; Buchanan, L.; Qian, Z.R.; Fuchs, C.S.; Lin, X.; et al. Clinical presentation, recurrence, and survival in patients with neuroendocrine tumors: Results from a prospective institutional database. *Endocr. Relat. Cancer* **2013**, *20*, 187–196. [CrossRef]
37. Kim, H.; Song, K.B.; Hwang, D.W.; Lee, J.H.; Shadi, A.; Kim, S.C. Time-trend and recurrence analysis of pancreatic neuroendocrine tumors. *Endocr. Connect.* **2019**, *8*, 1052–1060. [CrossRef] [PubMed]
38. Dong, D.H.; Zhang, X.F.; Lopez-Aguiar, A.G.; Poultsides, G.; Makris, E.; Rocha, F.; Kanji, Z.; Weber, S.; Fisher, A.; Fields, R.; et al. Resection of pancreatic neuroendocrine tumors: Defining patterns and time course of recurrence. *HPB (Oxford)* **2019**. [CrossRef] [PubMed]
39. Lou, F.; Sarkaria, I.; Pietanza, C.; Travis, W.; Roh, M.S.; Sica, G.; Healy, D.; Rusch, V.; Huang, J. Recurrence of pulmonary carcinoid tumors after resection: Implications for postoperative surveillance. *Ann. Thorac. Surg.* **2013**, *96*, 1156–1162. [CrossRef] [PubMed]
40. Ciment, A.; Gil, J.; Teirstein, A. Late recurrent pulmonary typical carcinoid tumor: Case report and review of the literature. *Mt. Sinai J. Med.* **2006**, *73*, 884–886. [PubMed]
41. Hamad, A.M.; Rizzardi, G.; Marulli, G.; Rea, F. Nodal recurrence of pulmonary carcinoid 30 years after primary resection. *J. Thorac. Oncol.* **2008**, *3*, 680–681. [CrossRef] [PubMed]
42. Pulvirenti, A.; Javed, A.A.; Landoni, L.; Jamieson, N.B.; Chou, J.F.; Miotto, M.; He, J.; Gonen, M.; Pea, A.; Tang, L.H.; et al. Multi-institutional Development and External Validation of a Nomogram to Predict Recurrence After Curative Resection of Pancreatic Neuroendocrine Tumors. *Ann. Surg.* **2019**. [CrossRef]
43. Slagter, A.E.; Ryder, D.; Chakrabarty, B.; Lamarca, A.; Hubner, R.A.; Mansoor, W.; O'Reilly, D.A.; Fulford, P.E.; Klümpen, H.J.; Valle, J.W.; et al. Prognostic factors for disease relapse in patients with neuroendocrine tumours who underwent curative surgery. *Surg. Oncol.* **2016**, *25*, 223–228. [CrossRef]
44. Zaidi, M.Y.; Lopez-Aguiar, A.G.; Switchenko, J.M.; Lipscomb, J.; Andreasi, V.; Partelli, S.; Gamboa, A.C.; Lee, R.M.; Poultsides, G.A.; Dillhoff, M.; et al. A Novel Validated Recurrence Risk Score to Guide a Pragmatic Surveillance Strategy After Resection of Pancreatic Neuroendocrine Tumors: An International Study of 1006 Patients. *Ann. Surg.* **2019**, *270*, 422–433. [CrossRef]
45. Cejas, P.; Drier, Y.; Dreijerink, K.M.A.; Brosens, L.A.A.; Deshpande, V.; Epstein, C.B.; Conemans, E.B.; Morsink, F.H.M.; Graham, M.K.; Valk, G.D.; et al. Enhancer signatures stratify and predict outcomes of non-functional pancreatic neuroendocrine tumors. *Nat. Med.* **2019**, *25*, 1260–1265. [CrossRef]
46. Ausania, F. Retrospective studies and pancreatic adenocarcinoma: How far can we backdate? *Ann. Surg.* **2015**, *261*, e84. [CrossRef]
47. Partelli, S.; Javed, A.A.; Andreasi, V.; He, J.; Muffatti, F.; Weiss, M.J.; Sessa, F.; La Rosa, S.; Doglioni, C.; Zamboni, G.; et al. The number of positive nodes accurately predicts recurrence after pancreaticoduodenectomy for nonfunctioning neuroendocrine neoplasms. *Eur. J. Surg. Oncol.* **2018**, *44*, 778–783. [CrossRef] [PubMed]
48. Zaidi, M.Y.; Lopez-Aguiar, A.G.; Dillhoff, M.; Beal, E.; Poultsides, G.; Makris, E.; Rocha, F.; Crown, A.; Idrees, K.; Marincola Smith, P.; et al. Prognostic Role of Lymph Node Positivity and Number of Lymph Nodes Needed for Accurately Staging Small Bowel Neuroendocrine Tumors. *JAMA Surg.* **2019**, *154*, 134–140. [CrossRef] [PubMed]
49. Cusumano, G.; Fournel, L.; Strano, S.; Damotte, D.; Charpentier, M.C.; Galia, A.; Terminella, A.; Nicolosi, M.; Regnard, J.F.; Alifano, M. Surgical Resection for Pulmonary Carcinoid: Long-Term Results of Multicentric Study-The Importance of Pathological N Status, More Than We Thought. *Lung* **2017**, *195*, 789–798. [CrossRef] [PubMed]
50. Hill, K.D.; Einstein, A.J. New approaches to reduce radiation exposure. *Trends Cardiovasc. Med.* **2016**, *26*, 55–65. [CrossRef] [PubMed]
51. Ramage, J.K.; Davies, A.H.; Ardill, J.; Bax, N.; Caplin, M.; Grossman, A.; Hawkins, R.; Mcnicol, A.M.; Reed, N.; Sutton, R.; et al. Guidelines for the management of gastroenteropancreatic neuroendocrine (including carcinoid) tumours. *Gut* **2005**, *54* (Suppl. 4), iv1–iv16. [CrossRef] [PubMed]
52. Garcia-Carbonero, R.; Vilardell, F.; Jimenez-Fonseca, P.; González-Campora, R.; González, E.; Cuatrecasas, M.; Capdevila, J.; Aranda, I.; Barriuso, J.; Matías-Guiu, X.; et al. Guidelines for biomarker testing in gastroenteropancreatic neuroendocrine neoplasms: A national consensus of the Spanish Society of Pathology and the Spanish Society of Medical Oncology. *Clin. Transl. Oncol.* **2014**, *16*, 243–256. [CrossRef] [PubMed]

53. Adaway, J.E.; Dobson, R.; Walsh, J.; Cuthbertson, D.J.; Monaghan, P.J.; Trainer, P.J.; Valle, J.W.; Keevil, B.G. Serum and plasma 5-hydroxyindoleacetic acid as an alternative to 24-h urine 5-hydroxyindoleacetic acid measurement. *Ann. Clin. Biochem.* **2016**, *53*, 554–560. [CrossRef] [PubMed]
54. Isgro, M.A.; Bottoni, P.; Scatena, R. Neuron-Specific Enolase as a Biomarker: Biochemical and Clinical Aspects. *Adv. Exp. Med. Biol.* **2015**, *867*, 125–143. [PubMed]
55. Bonato, M.; Cerati, M.; Pagani, A.; Papotti, M.; Bosi, F.; Bussolati, G.; Capella, C. Differential diagnostic patterns of lung neuroendocrine tumours. A clinico-pathological and immunohistochemical study of 122 cases. *Virchows Arch. A Pathol. Anat. Histopathol.* **1992**, *420*, 201–211. [CrossRef]
56. Gut, P.; Czarnywojtek, A.; Fischbach, J.; Bączyk, M.; Ziemnicka, K.; Wrotkowska, E.; Gryczyńska, M.; Ruchała, M. Chromogranin A—unspecific neuroendocrine marker. Clinical utility and potential diagnostic pitfalls. *Arch. Med. Sci.* **2016**, *12*, 1–9. [CrossRef]
57. Malczewska, A.; Witkowska, M.; Makulik, K.; Bocian, A.; Walter, A.; Pilch-Kowalczyk, J.; Zajęcki, W.; Bodei, L.; Oberg, K.E.; Kos-Kudła, B. NETest liquid biopsy is diagnostic of small intestine and pancreatic neuroendocrine tumors and correlates with imaging. *Endocr. Connect.* **2019**, *8*, 442–453. [CrossRef] [PubMed]
58. Malczewska, A.; Oberg, K.; Bodei, L.; Aslanian, H.; Lewczuk, A.; Filosso, P.L.; Wójcik-Giertuga, M.; Rydel, M.; Zielińska-Leś, I.; Walter, A.; et al. NETest Liquid Biopsy Is Diagnostic of Lung Neuroendocrine Tumors and Identifies Progressive Disease. *Neuroendocrinology* **2019**, *108*, 219–231. [CrossRef] [PubMed]
59. Oberg, K.; Krenning, E.; Sundin, A.; Aslanian, H.; Lewczuk, A.; Filosso, P.L.; Wójcik-Giertuga, M.; Rydel, M.; Zielińska-Leś, I.; Walter, A.; et al. A Delphic consensus assessment: Imaging and biomarkers in gastroenteropancreatic neuroendocrine tumor disease management. *Endocr. Connect.* **2016**, *5*, 174–187. [CrossRef] [PubMed]
60. Hemminki, K.; Li, X. Incidence trends and risk factors of carcinoid tumors: A nationwide epidemiologic study from Sweden. *Cancer* **2001**, *92*, 2204–2210. [CrossRef]
61. Basu, S.; Adnan, A. Well-differentiated grade 3 neuroendocrine tumours and poorly differentiated grade 3 neuroendocrine carcinomas: Will dual tracer PET-computed tomography (68Ga-DOTATATE and FDG) play a pivotal role in differentiation and guiding management strategies? *Nucl. Med. Commun.* **2019**, *40*, 1086–1087. [CrossRef]
62. Abgral, R.; Leboulleux, S.; Deandreis, D.; Aupérin, A.; Lumbroso, J.; Dromain, C.; Duvillard, P.; Elias, D.; de Baere, T.; Guigay, J.; et al. Performance of (18)fluorodeoxyglucose-positron emission tomography and somatostatin receptor scintigraphy for high Ki67 (>/=10%) well-differentiated endocrine carcinoma staging. *J. Clin. Endocrinol. Metab.* **2011**, *96*, 665–671. [CrossRef]
63. Park, C.M.; Goo, J.M.; Lee, H.J.; Kim, M.A.; Lee, C.H.; Kang, M.J. Tumors in the tracheobronchial tree: CT and FDG PET features. *Radiographics* **2009**, *29*, 55–71. [CrossRef]
64. Daniels, C.E.; Lowe, V.J.; Aubry, M.C.; Allen, M.S.; Jett, J.R. The utility of fluorodeoxyglucose positron emission tomography in the evaluation of carcinoid tumors presenting as pulmonary nodules. *Chest* **2007**, *131*, 255–260. [CrossRef]
65. Pattenden, H.A.; Leung, M.; Beddow, E.; Dusmet, M.; Nicholson, A.G.; Shackcloth, M.; Mohamed, S.; Darr, A.; Naidu, B.; Iyer, S.; et al. Test performance of PET-CT for mediastinal lymph node staging of pulmonary carcinoid tumours. *Thorax* **2015**, *70*, 379–381. [CrossRef]
66. Brabander, T.; Kwekkeboom, D.J.; Feelders, R.A.; Brouwers, A.H.; Teunissen, J.J. Nuclear Medicine Imaging of Neuroendocrine Tumors. *Front. Horm. Res.* **2015**, *44*, 73–87. [CrossRef]
67. Mojtahedi, A.; Thamake, S.; Tworowska, I.; Ranganathan, D.; Delpassand, E.S. The value of (68)Ga-DOTATATE PET/CT in diagnosis and management of neuroendocrine tumors compared to current FDA approved imaging modalities: A review of literature. *Am. J. Nucl. Med. Mol. Imaging* **2014**, *4*, 426–434. [PubMed]
68. Al-Nahhas, A.; Win, Z.; Szyszko, T.; Singh, A.; Nanni, C.; Fanti, S.; Rubello, D. Gallium-68 PET: A new frontier in receptor cancer imaging. *Anticancer Res.* **2007**, *27*, 4087–4094. [PubMed]
69. Breeman, W.A.; de, B.E.; Sze, C.H.; Konijnenberg, M.; Kwekkeboom, D.J.; Krenning, E.P. (68)Ga-labeled DOTA-peptides and (68)Ga-labeled radiopharmaceuticals for positron emission tomography: Current status of research, clinical applications, and future perspectives. *Semin. Nucl. Med.* **2011**, *41*, 314–321. [CrossRef] [PubMed]
70. Reubi, J.C.; Waser, B.; Liu, Q.; Laissue, J.A.; Schonbrunn, A. Subcellular distribution of somatostatin sst2A receptors in human tumors of the nervous and neuroendocrine systems: Membranous versus intracellular location. *J. Clin. Endocrinol. Metab.* **2000**, *85*, 3882–3891. [CrossRef] [PubMed]

71. Manoharan, P.N.S.; Lamarca, A.; Calero, J.; Chan, P.S.; Lopera Sierra, M.; Caplin, M.; Valle, J.W. Safety and Tolerability of "Ready-to-Use" (SOMAKIT TOC®) 68Ga-DOTA0-Tyr3-Octreotide (68Ga-DOTATOC) for Injection in Patients with Proven Gastro-Entero-Pancreatic Neuroendocrine Tumours (GEP-NETs). In Proceedings of the 14th Annual ENETS, Barcelona, Spain, 8–10 March 2017; Abstract Number 1759.
72. Hofmann, M.; Maecke, H.; Borner, R.; Weckesser, E.; Schöffski, P.; Oei, L.; Schumacher, J.; Henze, M.; Heppeler, A.; Meyer, J.; et al. Biokinetics and imaging with the somatostatin receptor PET radioligand (68)Ga-DOTATOC: Preliminary data. *Eur. J. Nucl. Med.* **2001**, *28*, 1751–1757. [CrossRef] [PubMed]
73. Kowalski, J.; Henze, M.; Schuhmacher, J.; Mäcke, H.R.; Hofmann, M.; Haberkorn, U. Evaluation of positron emission tomography imaging using [68Ga]-DOTA-D Phe(1)-Tyr(3)-Octreotide in comparison to [111In]-DTPAOC SPECT. First results in patients with neuroendocrine tumors. *Mol. Imaging Biol.* **2003**, *5*, 42–48. [CrossRef]
74. Gabriel, M.; Decristoforo, C.; Kendler, D.; Dobrozemsky, G.; Heute, D.; Uprimny, C.; Kovacs, P.; Von Guggenberg, E.; Bale, R.; Virgolini, I.J. 68Ga-DOTA-Tyr3-octreotide PET in neuroendocrine tumors: Comparison with somatostatin receptor scintigraphy and CT. *J. Nucl. Med.* **2007**, *48*, 508–518. [CrossRef] [PubMed]
75. Buchmann, I.; Henze, M.; Engelbrecht, S.; Eisenhut, M.; Runz, A.; Schäfer, M.; Schilling, T.; Haufe, S.; Herrmann, T.; Haberkorn, U. Comparison of 68Ga-DOTATOC PET and 111In-DTPAOC (Octreoscan) SPECT in patients with neuroendocrine tumours. *Eur. J. Nucl. Med. Mol. Imaging* **2007**, *34*, 1617–1626. [CrossRef] [PubMed]
76. Putzer, D.; Gabriel, M.; Henninger, B.; Kendler, D.; Uprimny, C.; Dobrozemsky, G.; Decristoforo, C.; Bale, R.J.; Jaschke, W.; Virgolini, I.J. Bone metastases in patients with neuroendocrine tumor: 68Ga-DOTA-Tyr3-octreotide PET in comparison to CT and bone scintigraphy. *J. Nucl. Med.* **2009**, *50*, 1214–1221. [CrossRef]
77. Srirajaskanthan, R.; Kayani, I.; Quigley, A.M.; Soh, J.; Caplin, M.E.; Bomanji, J. The role of 68Ga-DOTATATE PET in patients with neuroendocrine tumors and negative or equivocal findings on 111In-DTPA-octreotide scintigraphy. *J. Nucl. Med.* **2010**, *51*, 875–882. [CrossRef]
78. Lamarca, A.; Pritchard, D.M.; Westwood, T.; Papaxoinis, G.; Nonaka, D.; Vinjamuri, S.; Valle, J.W.; Manoharan, P.; Mansoor, W. 68Gallium DOTANOC-PET Imaging in Lung Carcinoids: Impact on Patients' Management. *Neuroendocrinology* **2018**, *106*, 128–138. [CrossRef]
79. Geijer, H.; Breimer, L.H. Somatostatin receptor PET/CT in neuroendocrine tumours: Update on systematic review and meta-analysis. *Eur. J. Nucl. Med. Mol. Imaging* **2013**, *40*, 1770–1780. [CrossRef] [PubMed]
80. Sharma, P.; Arora, S.; Karunanithi, S.; Khadgawat, R.; Durgapal, P.; Sharma, R.; Kandasamy, D.; Bal, C.; Kumar, R. Somatostatin receptor based PET/CT imaging with 68Ga-DOTA-Nal3-octreotide for localization of clinically and biochemically suspected insulinoma. *Q. J. Nucl. Med. Mol. Imaging* **2016**, *60*, 69–76.
81. Wild, D.; Bomanji, J.B.; Benkert, P.; Maecke, H.; Ell, P.J.; Reubi, J.C.; Caplin, M.E. Comparison of 68Ga-DOTANOC and 68Ga-DOTATATE PET/CT within patients with gastroenteropancreatic neuroendocrine tumors. *J. Nucl. Med.* **2013**, *54*, 364–372. [CrossRef]
82. Ambrosini, V.; Campana, D.; Bodei, L.; Nanni, C.; Castellucci, P.; Allegri, V.; Montini, G.C.; Tomassetti, P.; Paganelli, G.; Fanti, S. 68Ga-DOTANOC PET/CT clinical impact in patients with neuroendocrine tumors. *J. Nucl. Med.* **2010**, *51*, 669–673. [CrossRef] [PubMed]
83. Naswa, N.; Sharma, P.; Soundararajan, R.; Karunanithi, S.; Nazar, A.H.; Kumar, R.; Malhotra, A.; Bal, C. Diagnostic performance of somatostatin receptor PET/CT using 68Ga-DOTANOC in gastrinoma patients with negative or equivocal CT findings. *Abdom. Imaging* **2013**, *38*, 552–560. [CrossRef] [PubMed]
84. Ilhan, H.; Fendler, W.P.; Cyran, C.C.; Spitzweg, C.; Auernhammer, C.J.; Gildehaus, F.J.; Bartenstein, P.; Angele, M.K.; Haug, A.R. Impact of (68)Ga-DOTATATE PET/CT on the surgical management of primary neuroendocrine tumors of the pancreas or ileum. *Ann. Surg. Oncol.* **2015**, *22*, 164–171. [CrossRef]
85. Kayani, I.; Conry, B.G.; Groves, A.M.; Win, T.; Dickson, J.; Caplin, M.; Bomanji, J.B. A comparison of 68Ga-DOTATATE and 18F-FDG PET/CT in pulmonary neuroendocrine tumors. *J. Nucl. Med.* **2009**, *50*, 1927–1932. [CrossRef]

86. Bodei, L.; Ambrosini, V.; Herrmann, K.; Modlin, I. Current Concepts in (68)Ga-DOTATATE Imaging of Neuroendocrine Neoplasms: Interpretation, Biodistribution, Dosimetry, and Molecular Strategies. *J. Nucl. Med.* **2017**, *58*, 1718–1726. [CrossRef]
87. Haug, A.R.; Cindea-Drimus, R.; Auernhammer, C.J.; Reincke, M.; Beuschlein, F.; Wängler, B.; Uebleis, C.; Schmidt, G.P.; Spitzweg, C.; Bartenstein, P.; et al. Neuroendocrine tumor recurrence: Diagnosis with 68Ga-DOTATATE PET/CT. *Radiology* **2014**, *270*, 517–525. [CrossRef]

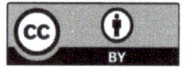 © 2019 by the authors. Licensee MDPI, Basel, Switzerland. This article is an open access article distributed under the terms and conditions of the Creative Commons Attribution (CC BY) license (http://creativecommons.org/licenses/by/4.0/).

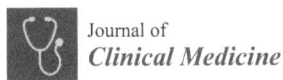

Review

Updates on the Role of Molecular Alterations and NOTCH Signalling in the Development of Neuroendocrine Neoplasms

Claudia von Arx [1,2,†], Monica Capozzi [1,†], Elena López-Jiménez [3,†], Alessandro Ottaiano [4], Fabiana Tatangelo [5], Annabella Di Mauro [5], Guglielmo Nasti [4], Maria Lina Tornesello [6,*,‡] and Salvatore Tafuto [1,*,‡] On behalf of ENETs (European NeuroEndocrine Tumor Society) Center of Excellence of Naples, Italy

1. Department of Abdominal Oncology, Istituto Nazionale Tumori, IRCCS Fondazione "G. Pascale", 80131 Naples, Italy
2. Department of Surgery and Cancer, Imperial College London, London W12 0HS, UK
3. Cancer Cell Metabolism Group. Centre for Haematology, Immunology and Inflammation Department, Imperial College London, London W12 0HS, UK
4. SSD Innovative Therapies for Abdominal Metastases—Department of Abdominal Oncology, Istituto Nazionale Tumori, IRCCS—Fondazione "G. Pascale", 80131 Naples, Italy
5. Department of Pathology, Istituto Nazionale Tumori, IRCCS—Fondazione "G. Pascale", 80131 Naples, Italy
6. Unit of Molecular Biology and Viral Oncology, Department of Research, Istituto Nazionale Tumori IRCCS Fondazione Pascale, 80131 Naples, Italy
* Correspondence: m.tornesello@istitutotumori.na.it (M.L.T.); s.tafuto@istitutotumori.na.it (S.T.)
† The authors are the co-first of this study.
‡ The authors are the co-last of this study.

Received: 10 July 2019; Accepted: 20 August 2019; Published: 22 August 2019

Abstract: Neuroendocrine neoplasms (NENs) comprise a heterogeneous group of rare malignancies, mainly originating from hormone-secreting cells, which are widespread in human tissues. The identification of mutations in ATRX/DAXX genes in sporadic NENs, as well as the high burden of mutations scattered throughout the multiple endocrine neoplasia type 1 (MEN-1) gene in both sporadic and inherited syndromes, provided new insights into the molecular biology of tumour development. Other molecular mechanisms, such as the NOTCH signalling pathway, have shown to play an important role in the pathogenesis of NENs. NOTCH receptors are expressed on neuroendocrine cells and generally act as tumour suppressor proteins, but in some contexts can function as oncogenes. The biological heterogeneity of NENs suggests that to fully understand the role and the potential therapeutic implications of gene mutations and NOTCH signalling in NENs, a comprehensive analysis of genetic alterations, NOTCH expression patterns and their potential role across all NEN subtypes is required.

Keywords: neuroendocrine neoplasms; NOTCH; cancer-driven genes; mutational mechanism; germline mutations; small cell lung carcinoma; pancreatic NET; small bowel NET; medullary thyroid carcinoma; malignant castration-resistant prostatic cells

1. Introduction

Neuroendocrine cells are sensor cells, which play an important role in the connection between the nervous system and endocrine organs. In response to neurogenic stimulation, neuroendocrine cells secrete several molecules, including peptide hormones, which produce slow and long-lasting effects. Neuroendocrine cells are widely scattered throughout the human body. They are present in the gastro-entero-pancreatic tract, uro-genital apparatus, lung, breast and skin, as well as in the central and peripheral nervous system. These cells are able to dedifferentiate and transdifferentiate under physiological conditions in response to intracellular metabolic pathways and microenvironmental stress conditions [1].

NOTCH signaling is a highly conserved cell-signaling pathway that is implicated in different stages of development through the regulation of cell proliferation, differentiation and cell death.

In the neuroendocrine system, NOTCH signaling drives the maturation process of multi-potent cells to become functionally competent cells during the early stage of embryonic neuroendocrine development [2]. For instance, NOTCH signaling regulates the ductal and endocrine differentiation of pancreatic cells during the development of the pancreas [3].

Neuroendocrine neoplasms (NENs) are originated from the neoplastic transformation of neuroendocrine cells at various anatomic locations, with the gastrointestinal tract, the endocrine pancreas and the respiratory tract being the most involved sites. [4].

Little is known about the mechanisms of oncogenic transformation and metastatic dissemination of neuroendocrine cells, but it is known that despite some common molecular characteristics, NENs originating in different organs have distinct signatures and display significant biological heterogeneity.

In this heterogeneous neoplastic setting, the NOTCH pathway has shown to have a role by triggering both tumour suppressor and oncogenic functions in some neuroendocrine cell lines and in different subtypes of NENs [5–10].

The availability of treatments with a modulatory activity on NOTCH-dependent pathways, and the possibility to use the molecular alterations as diagnostic and prognostic markers, has highlighted the need of a deeper knowledge on the NOTCH pathway role and the different molecular signatures in NENs.

This review will summarize the current knowledge on the molecular heterogeneity of NENs and the complex function of NOTCH signalling in different types of NENs, as well as the new therapeutic approaches based on NOTCH pathway modulation.

2. Neuroendocrine Neoplasms and Molecular Heterogeneity

Neuroendocrine neoplasms are genomically and clinically heterogeneous. This heterogeneity occurs between cancers originating from different organs, within the cancers originating in the same organ, and between primary and metastatic lesions [4,11–13]. For instance, small intestine NENs are genomic stable cancers, with a low mutational load compared with NENs originated from different organs, such as the lung and pancreas. Viral-associated Merkel carcinomas have a low mutational burden, in contrast to ultraviolet (UV)-induced Merkel cell carcinomas [14]. The full understanding of the molecular mechanisms and the clinical significance of this heterogeneity could lead to the identification of new hallmarks to target in the neuroendocrine neoplasms' treatment.

Current advances in genomic analysis techniques have enabled to identify recurrent mutations and chromosomal aberrations at the base of the molecular landscape of NENs [15,16].

Recurrent mutations have been identified in multiple endocrine neoplasia type 1 (*MEN1*) and von Hippel–Lindau (*VHL*) genes, in chromatin remodelling genes, such as *DAXX* and *ATRX*, in mechanistic target of rapamycin (mTOR) pathway genes, especially in phosphatase and tensin homolog (*PTEN*), tuberous sclerosis complex 2 (*TSC2*), and phosphatidylinositol-4,5-bisphosphate 3-kinase catalytic subunit alpha (*PIK3CA*), in checkpoint kinase 2 (*CHEK2*) tumour suppressor gene, in telomerase maintenance genes, in the cell cycle regulator cyclin dependent kinase inhibitor 1B (*CDKN1B*) and in the DNA repair gene mutY DNA glycosylase (*MUTYH*) [15,16]. These mutations can occur in genetic syndromes, such as multiple endocrine neoplasia type 1 (MEN1), tuberous sclerosis complex (TSC1/2), neurofibromatosis type 1 (NF1), and von Hippel–Lindau (VHL) syndrome, or in sporadic NENs, and can be germline or somatic mutations [15–17]. Genetic syndromes account for 15–20% of NENs, while the remaining 80–85% are sporadic.

Interestingly, as confirmation of the high heterogeneity of NENs, whole exome sequencing analysis performed in different studies has identified only 21 genes commonly altered between the small intestinal NENs samples analysed from different patients [11,18]. Furthermore, comparing the results of these studies on small bowel NENs with the one on pancreatic NENs, a concordance of only 17 genes with somatic mutations was found [11,15,18].

In addition, some mutations, namely mutations in *MEN1* and *DAXX/ATRX* genes, are associated with a better prognosis, and they seem to occur very rarely in poorly differentiated neuroendocrine carcinomas (NECs) [19]. On the other hand, mutation in *TP53*, *RB1*, *PTEN* and *PIK3CA* are more frequent in poorly differentiated NECs [19,20].

In the following paragraph, we summarise the current knowledge and the clinical significance of the most common genetic alterations in NENs, classifying them according to their hereditary or sporadic condition.

3. Common Genetic Alterations and Molecular Pathways in the Development of Neuroendocrine Neoplasms

3.1. Heritable Genetic Traits in Neuroendocrine Neoplasms

NENs comprise at least ten recognized inherited NEN syndromes, including multiple endocrine neoplasia type 1 and 2 (MEN-1 and MEN-2), von Hippel–Lindau syndrome (VHL) and neurofibromatosis type 1 (NF1) [21].

MEN-1 is a rare autosomal dominant syndrome caused by inactivating mutations in the MEN-1 gene, and mostly associated with the appearance of neoplastic lesions in the pancreas and duodenum, as well as in pituitary and parathyroid glands [22,23]. The majority of germline mutations in the MEN-1 gene cause the truncation or absence of the menin protein in cancer cells. Typically, tumour development is associated with the mutation of both MEN-1 alleles, however, an incomplete inactivation of this gene has been observed in thymic and duodenal NETs [24,25]. The menin protein is usually located in the nucleus, cytoplasm and around telomeres. However, its specific biological role has not yet been described [26].

MEN-2 syndrome is an inherited autosomal dominant disorder comprising MEN-2A (55% of all cases), MEN-2B (5–10%) and familial medullary thyroid carcinoma (FMTC; 35–40%) [27]. The MEN-2A and MEN-2B patients have almost 100% risk of developing MTC and about 50% risk of developing pheochromocytoma and parathyroid adenomas. MEN-2 syndrome is caused by mutations in RET proto-oncogene, encoding a tyrosine kinase receptor. These mutations cause activation of RAS/MAPK (mitogen-activated protein kinases) and PI3K/AKT (phosphatidylinositol 3-kinase/Protein Kinase B) signalling pathways [28] and may occur in two different regions of the RET gene, originating two different types of disorders. In addition, the familial MTC (FMTC) syndrome, which is also caused by RET mutations, is only associated with MTC, but is less aggressive than MEN-2 tumours [29].

MEN-4 is a rare autosomal dominant syndrome predisposed to NETs development, such as parathyroid and pituitary adenomas, associated with the germline mutations in CDKN1B genes encoding the p27kip protein [30]. However, more studies are needed to know the penetrance and biological effect of CDKN1B mutations in these patients.

Von Hippel–Lindau (VHL) syndrome is associated with pheochromocytomas, paragangliomas and pancreatic neoplasia, and is caused by the loss of the VHL tumour suppressor gene, regulating the hypoxia-inducible factor (HIF) and vascular endothelial growth factor (VEGF) pathways [31–33]. The VHL protein shuttles between the nucleus and cytoplasm, binding to elongen C, elongen B, Cullin-2 (Cul2), and RING-box protein 1 (Rbx1) and degrading the alpha subunits of HIF in an oxygen-dependent manner [32,34,35]. Lack of degradation of this factor due to the absence of the VHL protein results, for instance, in an uncontrolled production of factors promoting blood vessel formation (e.g., VEGF) and is implicated in tumour development. The germline mutations in the VHL gene are extremely heterogeneous and are spread throughout the coding sequence. They are present in virtually all families with VHL syndrome, although the exact molecular mechanism of development of NETs in VHL has still many unknowns [36].

Neurofibromatosis type 1 (NF1) syndrome is another familiar neuroendocrine tumour (NET) disorder, which is associated with duodenal NETs or pheochromocytomas and is linked to RAS and ERK/MAPK pathways' deregulations [37]. Genetic alterations of the NF1 gene include missense, nonsense and splice site mutations, as well as insertions/deletions (in/dels) and chromosomal rearrangements [38]. Tuberosclerosis gene TSC1 (9q34) and TSC2 (16p13.3) are regulated by neurofibromin through mTOR activation, linking the three proteins in terms of their potential roles in tumour progression [37].

Loss of function of the NF1 gene causes mTOR activation and tumour development. Disruption of TSC2 in pancreatic beta cells induces beta cell mass expansion in an mTOR-dependent manner [39]. Furthermore, it has recently been demonstrated that patients with pancreatic NET (pNET), and loss of PTEN protein, as well as tuberosclerosis 1 protein, show a significantly shorter survival [40].

Familial pheochromocytoma and paraganglioma syndromes are autosomal-dominant disorders caused mostly by germline mutations in the succinate dehydrogenase subunit (SDH) genes, such as SDHB, SDHC, SDHD, SDHA, and SDHAF2 (succinate dehydrogenase complex assembly factor 2). These are encoding factors required for the assembly of the mitochondrial complex II [32,33,41–50]. This mitochondrial complex participates in two main cellular processes: the Krebs cycle and the electron-transport chain. The mutations in the key components for the formation of complex II decrease the enzymatic activity of the rest of the complex. The link between the perturbation in complex II and tumorigenesis still has many unknowns. SDH deficiency leads to pseudohypoxic conditions in cancer cells. However, this fact alone is probably not sufficient to induce the tumorigenic process, and thus different possibilities appear to be feasible; for instance, the implication of ROS or the possibility of the inhibition of other α-ketoglutarate-dependent enzymes.

SDH mutations are commonly associated with multiple pheochromocytomas and paragangliomas. However, gastrointestinal stromal tumours, SDH-deficient renal cell carcinoma and pituitary adenomas can also be associated with these mutations [51,52].

3.2. Genetic Alterations and Tumour Mutation Burden in NENs

Several chromosomal alterations and gene mutations have been consistently identified in different types of sporadic NENs, although the tumour mutational burden is relatively low compared to other tumour types [21]. In fact, massive parallel sequencing showed that only 24 cancer driver genes are affected by non-synonymous mutations in neuroendocrine neoplasms [53]. Remarkably, cancer driver genes and mutations are unevenly distributed in different tumour types and may contribute to the mechanisms of NEN heterogeneity. The factors encoded by these mutated genes may affect several pathways involved in cell proliferation, metabolism and chromatin modification.

The genetic landscape of gastro-entero-pancreatic neuroendocrine neoplasms (GEP-NENs) confirmed the essential differences of mutational profiles between well-differentiated NETs, including those with a high proliferation index, and NECs [54].

Mutations in TP53 and RB1 genes are pivotal drivers in poorly differentiated NECs of any anatomical origin [16,55–58]. Mutations in the TP53 gene have been consistently detected in poorly-differentiated GEP-NECs, with a frequency ranging from 20% to 73% of the tested patients [20,55,59,60]. The presence of TP53 mutations in GEP-NECs correlates with poor survival [20], and recently Ali et al. have demonstrated that p53 immunoexpression in colorectal NECs correlates with a poorer response to platinum-based chemotherapy and worse prognosis [61]. These results suggest a potential diagnostic, prognostic and predictive role of p53 immunoexpression in GEP-NECs, one that is currently under investigation in different trials.

The inactivation of RB1 gene product, which occurs mainly by somatic mutations, has been reported in 71% of poorly differentiated pancreatic NECs [54].

KRAS mutations have been identified in gastric, pancreatic and colorectal NECs with frequencies ranging from 8% to 60% [20,54,60,62–66].

On the other hand, BRAF mutations were only found in colorectal NECs with a frequency between 13% and 59% [67], as well as APC affecting some cancer cases [68].

The genetic alterations characterizing poorly differentiated NECs are absent in Grade (G) 3 NETs. This subtype presents typical mutations of G1/G2 NETs. For example, G3 pancreatic NETs showed high frequency of MEN1, DAXX, and ATRX mutations or protein loss (31–44%, 9–25% and 18–36%, respectively). DAXX and ATRX mutations also significantly correlate with the presence of mutations in mTOR regulators and were associated with poor prognosis in the G2 NETs [16]. Therefore, the scientific community is proposing these mutations as possible biomarkers to distinguish G3 pancreatic NETs from NECs [69]. This has a particular clinical relevance, due to the fact that NECs and G3 NETs are detected at an advanced stage.

The molecular similarities between G1/G2 and G3 NETs suggested a new model for GEP-NEN tumorigenesis in which poorly differentiated NECs and well-differentiated NETs, including G3 NETs, were originated from a common-normal neuroendocrine progenitor through different routes [70]. These foresee the alteration of TP53 and RB1 for all poorly-differentiated NECs, and specific alterations for well-differentiated pancreatic NETs and small intestine NETs [71].

Despite the remarkable biological heterogeneity of NETs, the mammalian target of rapamycin (mTOR) molecular pathway has been found to be prominently altered in a vast majority of NETs [72]. mTOR is a kinase-dependent signalling cascade, formed by the mammalian target of rapamycin complex 1 and 2 (mTORC1 and mTORC2), whose main function is related to controlling cell growth. Mutations in NF1, TSC2 or PTEN-encoding for key suppressor genes of this pathway, and altered expression of the mTOR pathway components, are common hallmarks of a great proportion of NETs, wherein these alterations seem to be directly related with tumour development and progression [72].

Recent evidence pointed out a key role of the NOTCH signalling pathway in NEN development, progression and heterogeneity [73]. Loss-of-function mutations in NOTCH family genes, particularly in NOTCH1, have been identified in human and mouse small cell lung cancer (SCLC) and in neuroendocrine pancreatic cells [58,74]. The integrity of NOTCH components is very important for the proper signalling transduction across the pathway. The canonical Notch cascade needs to receive a signal and be able to act in a ligand-receptor manner for communicating the signal inside the cells. This signal translocation promotes several transcriptional changes in the cellular program that allow cells to perform different functions. With an obstacle on this cell signalling cascade, the cells have to deal with unexpected changes in their programs, usually due to different mutations that interfere in the adequate cell–cell communication or in the transcriptional regulation within the cell.

For a better understanding on how these genetic mutations or genomic alterations could lead to the development of neuroendocrine tumours, in the following section, the composition of NOTCH receptors and the main elements involved in the NOTCH signalling transduction will be explained in detail.

4. Structure of NOTCH Receptors and the NOTCH Signalling Pathway

The NOTCH receptor family in mammals comprises four transmembrane proteins (NOTCH1–4), which are evolutionarily conserved with a high homology between different species. NOTCH receptors are activated by trans-ligands expressed on neighbouring cells, whereas cis-ligands within the same cell inhibit the NOTCH signalling [75].

The four NOTCH receptor isoforms in mammals are characterized by an extracellular region of repetitive epidermal growth factor (EGF)-like sequences, which are involved in the interaction with delta-like ligands (DLL1, DLL3, DLL4) and jagged proteins (JAG1, JAG2), by a negative regulatory region (NRR) that prevents Notch activation in the absence of the correct signal, by a single transmembrane portion and by an intra-cytoplasmic tail involved in the signal transduction (Figure 1). The number of EGF-like repeats varies between the four NOTCH receptors, being 36 for NOTCH-1 and 2 receptors, 34 for NOTCH-3 and 29 for NOTCH-4. The NRR consists of three cysteine-rich LIN12-NOTCH repeats (LNR) and a heterodimerization domain (HD). The intracellular domain is composed of a recombining binding protein suppressor of hairless (RBPj) associate module, ankirin repeats (ANK) and a C-terminal region rich in proline (P), glutamine (E), serine (S) and threonine (T) residues (PEST). S2 and S3 regions are, respectively, the metalloprotease and γ-secretase sites of cleavage. The expression of these receptors is in a cell- and tissue-type specific manner.

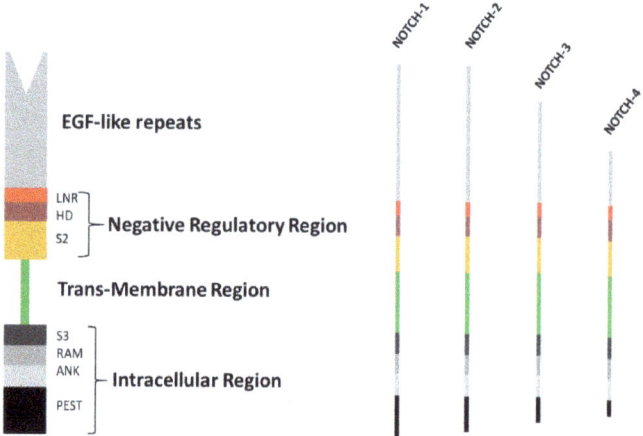

Figure 1. Structure of four human NOTCH receptors: NOTCH receptors are composed of an extracellular region of repetitive epidermal growth factor (EGF)-like sequences (29–36 repeats), a negative regulatory region, a single transmembrane portion and an intra-cytoplasmic tail involved in signal transduction. S2 and S3 are, respectively, the metalloprotease and γ-secretase sites of cleavage. EGF: epidermal growth factor; LNR: cysteine-rich LIN12-NOTCH repeats; HD: heterodimerization domain; RAM: recombining binding protein suppressor of hairless (RBPJ) associate module; ANK: ankyrin repeats; PEST: region rich in proline (P), glutamine (E), serine (S) and threonine (T) residues.

The interaction between NOTCH receptors and their ligands initiates proteolytic cleavage of the receptor by a disintegrin and metalloprotease (ADAM). A subsequent cleavage by γ-secretase complex releases the NOTCH intracellular domain (NICD) of the receptor. NOTCH-NICD migrates into the nucleus where it binds to the recombining binding protein suppressor of hairless (RBPJ) and Mastermind-like (MAML) co-activators to assemble an active transcription complex on NOTCH-responsive genes (Figure 2).

Genes regulated by the NOTCH signalling pathway include the hairy-enhancer of split (Hes1, Hey1, Hey2) encoding the double-helical transcription factors with negative regulatory function, as well as c-Myc and cyclin D involved in cell cycle regulation [76].

The main roles of NOTCH have been associated with the regulation of homeostasis and cell proliferation, as well as the development and cell differentiation in a variety of tissues. This regulation can occur during both embryonic stages and postnatal life.

The plethora of ligands regulating NOTCH receptors have been extensively studied in different tumour types because of their onco-regulatory effects [77–79]. Depending on the biological microenvironment, the activation of NOTCH signalling seems to have a dual role, showing an oncogenic activity in certain tissues (i.e., the non-neuroendocrine component of small cell lung cancer) [73,80], and tumour-suppressor function in others (i.e., medullary thyroid carcinoma, small cell lung cancer, pancreatic and biliary neuroendocrine tumours) [81–84].

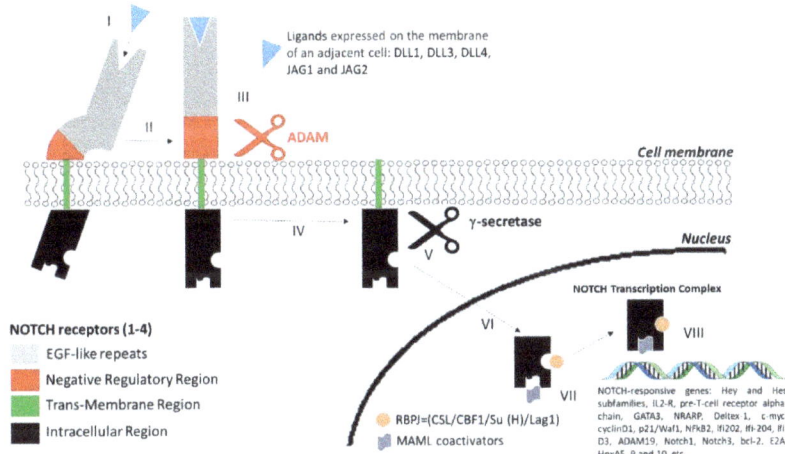

Figure 2. Schematic representation of NOTCH signalling pathway: Sequential steps in the NOTCH signalling pathway are shown as follows: I: NOTCH receptor binding to specific ligands; II: conformational change of the receptor; III: ADAMs-mediated cleavage; IV: recognition of the intracellular region by γ-secretase; V: γ-secretase mediated cleavage; VI: nuclear translocation; VII: binding to RBPJ and MAML; VIII: transcriptional activation DLL: delta-like ligands; JAG: jagged protein; ADAM: a disintegrin and metalloprotease; RBPJ: recombining binding protein suppressor of hairless; MAML: Mastermind-like co-activators.

5. The Role of NOTCH Signalling in NENs

Pre-clinical studies showed a heterogeneous expression of the NOTCH receptor family in tumoral tissues, and genome sequencing analysis has identified several NOTCH gene mutations in various solid and hematological malignancies [82,85–87].

The main role attributed to the NOTCH signalling pathway is as a mediator of cell differentiation. Depending on the NOTCH receptor expression levels, the cross-talk with other signalling pathways and the cellular context, NOTCH signalling can have an oncogenic or tumour suppressor role [85]. In addition, alterations of the NOTCH signalling pathway are responsible for the smooth transition from a non-neuroendocrine to a neuroendocrine phenotype, as a result of a coordinated anti-cancer drug response in pathological cell conditions.

Therefore, to understand completely the impact that NOTCH operates in the development of neuroendocrine tumours, the analysis of NOTCH signalling at different layers of genomic regulation is required, ranging from gene expression levels to epigenetic alterations, and involving its diverse components as NOTCH receptors and ligands.

In the biggest cancer killers, the study of the NOTCH pathway was a milestone, and several analyses elucidated its role in pathogenesis. The expression of the different isoforms was exanimated and the presence of mutations was assessed.

In breast cancer tissue, aberrant high levels of NOTCH1 and NOTCH2 were found in comparison with control tissue [88]. Moreover, alterations in Notch signalling were also linked to triple-negative breast cancer (TNBC). Mutations were found in NOTCH1–3 at the C-terminal PEST domain, and also in the prolyl-isomerase PIN1 (peptidylprolyl cis/trans isomarase, NIMA-interacting 1) [89], supporting the theory of the involvement of Notch in breast cancer.

In some neoplasms, mutation can contribute to enhance the physiological function of the pathway, as was described in a previous non-small cell lung carcinoma (NSCLC) analysis. In this study, it was demonstrated that the presence of a C-terminal mutation in the NOTCH-1 gene confers a gain of function, increasing the receptor signalling transduction in NSCLC cancer [90].

In colorectal cancer (CRC), the genomic alteration in the NOTCH pathway correlates with clinical outcome—it may lead cells to proliferate without differentiation or to maintain the transcriptional program of normal adult colon cells. A common upregulation of the NOTCH-1 gene expression was found in tumoral samples belonging to the three different CRC transcriptional subtypes, characterized by specific transcriptional programs related to the normal adult colon, early colon embryonic development and epithelial mesenchymal transition. This finding is consistent with the critical role of Notch pathway in CRC initiation [91].

Interestingly, a recent study showed that mutation of NOTCH1 in oral squamous cell carcinoma occurs in 15% of the Caucasian population, whereas in the Asian population the rate of NOTCH1 mutations was about 50% [92]. This finding emphasizes the need to clarify the NOTCH alteration prevalence in human cancer, even more in rare neoplasms.

In NENs, the NOTCH mutational status assessment has been analysed in only a few studies, conducing whole-genome sequencing in specific neuroendocrine neoplasms.

An up-to-date one next generation sequence study was performed on the small cell neuroendocrine carcinoma of uterine cervix (SCNEC). Deyin Xing et al., found oncogenic driver mutations in KRAS, Erb-B2, c-Myc, BCL6 and NOTCH1 in a cohort of 10 small-cell neuroendocrine carcinomas (SCNEC) of the uterine cervix, a rare but extremely aggressive tumour [93]. In addition, in a cohort of large cells, neuroendocrine carcinoma (LCNEC), the most relevant molecular alteration, was detected in DLL3, a well-known NOTCH canonical ligand. The DLL3 inhibition, in combination with the use of immunotherapy, has also been pointed out as a therapeutic option for LCNEC [94]. A separate study conducted whole-genome sequencing of small cell lung cancer (SCLC), identifying inactivating mutations in the NOTCH family genes in 25% of cases [58,95].

In the following paragraphs, we summarize the current knowledge on the epigenetic modifications and NOTCH signalling pathway alteration in different types of NENs.

5.1. NOTCH in NENs: The Epigenetic Implications

It is conceivable to think of epigenetic changes contributing to the pathological development of tissue and how these alterations could affect gene expression after stem cell differentiation, as happens in other neoplasms. The epigenetic modifications by definition encompass all the mechanisms that modify the genetic expression and alter the genome stability, without modifying the DNA sequence. These alterations not only can occur at the chromatin level and involve acetylation and deacetylation of the histones and the methylation of the cytosine at DNA level, but can also be caused by other molecules, such as non-coding RNAs, for instance, and long non-coding RNAs and microRNAs.

Experimental data suggests that epigenetic alterations are involved in neuroendocrine tumorigenesis [96,97]. Some pivotal preclinical studies were conducted to explore the role of epigenetic alterations in NETs, obtaining interesting results—silencing regulatory genes (Wnt signaling components) and aberrant mutations in core pathways contributes in NET pathogenesis [97]. Furthermore, missense mutation in the mixed-lineage leukemia protein 3 (MLL3) often triggers aggressive neuroendocrine tumours, medulloblastomas and Merkel cell carcinoma [98] by means of inducing genomic instability.

Moreover, lysine-specific histone demethylase 1A (LSD1) inhibitor ORY-1001 was described in small cell lung cancer (SCLC) because of its anti-tumorigenic role. This inhibitor activates the NOTCH pathway, inhibiting, consequently, the transcription factor achaete–scute complex-like 1 (ASCL1), with this ultimately leading to tumorigenesis repression and to the reversion of the neuroendocrine phenotype in this type of tumour. A complete and long-term tumour regression was obtained after treating with ORY-1001 SCLC patient-derived xenograft (PDX) mice models [99]. Thus, this inhibitor has been suggested as a potential new targeted therapy for SCLC.

Recent findings on the transcriptional activation of NOTCH appear to be regulated by means of microRNAs (miRNAs), small single-stranded RNAs that regulate gene expression post-transcriptionally. Preliminary research about how aberrant miRNA expression can influence neuroendocrine cell behaviours showed a direct post-transcriptional repression of NOTCH2 and RBPJ proteins operated by miR-375 (microRNA 375) in Merkel cell carcinoma (MCC), a rare cutaneous neuroendocrine malignancy [100]. This small molecule is having an increasing connotation in the modern pathology of NEN. Arvidsson et al. discovered that miR-375 is highly expressed in small intestinal neuroendocrine tumours and could be used as prognostic biomarker for survival [101].

In the age of precision medicine, the identification of epigenetic biomarkers in a subpopulation of patients could help clinicians to choose the most appropriate therapeutic strategy. Recently, epigenetic drugs are providing promising results in preclinical phases, making attractive the idea of their use in combination with standard chemotherapy or immunotherapy. However, further validation in clinical trials is needed, and side effects have to be assessed for the possible use of these combined strategies [102].

Currently, only a few studies have focused on the epigenetic landscape in NET, and even less if we point out the implications that may occur between these epigenetic factors and the NOTCH pathway. A coordinated effort between multidisciplinary groups of experts is needed to clarify the role of NOTCH in diverse neuroendocrine neoplasms.

In the following section, we summarize the evidence gathered to date on the role of the NOTCH signalling pathway in different NENs.

5.2. Role of NOTCH in Neuroendocrine Tumour of the Lung

In lung tissue, the role of NOTCH has been established as driving the differentiation of neuroendocrine cells present in the organ. NOTCH mutation can provoke a dysfunction of its activity and induce neuroendocrine differentiation from no-neuroendocrine progenitors. Clinical data indicate that some neuroendocrine neoplasms of the lung could relapse and present a secondary tumour formation after anticancer therapy.

Recent findings suggest that the presence of inactivating mutations in NOTCH signalling is involved in the pathogenesis of neuroendocrine neoplasms of the lung, being defined as more than 25% of the cases for small cell lung carcinomas (SCLC) [58,103]. This fact suggests that NOTCH signalling needs to be inactivated for the development of SCLC. Moreover, NOTCH signalling is involved in the modulation of the neural and neuroendocrine differentiation process that could mean the implication of mutations in NOTCH in the neuroendocrine features of these tumours, and also in disease progression and relapse.

NOTCH pathway deregulation has been also pointed out to have a role in chemoresistance in SCLC. The effect of NOTCH in tumorigenesis seems to be done throughout the activation of the delta-like protein 3 (DLL3). Its expression is directly correlated with ASCL1 transcription factor that was found expressed in 85% of SCLCs, in contrast with an absent or minimal expression in normal lung tissue. The overexpression of DLL3 in comparison with normal tissue was also found in primary patients' biopsies, as previously described Saunders et al. [104].

One of the features that differentiate DLL3 from other Notch ligands is its location in the Golgi that makes DLL3 able to interact with Notch1 and DLL1, blocking their transport to the endosomes for elimination and preventing them from reaching the cell surface and therefore preventing NOTCH activation. DLL3 appears to act as an inhibitor of the Notch receptor pathway.

In the mixed forms of small cell carcinomas, the modulation of the NOTCH system demonstrated the importance of this pathway in tumorigenesis and response to treatment—the activation of NOTCH reduces the particularly aggressive neuroendocrine subtype by increasing the epithelial component with a slower cell proliferation rate whose growth can be controlled with chemotherapy [73].

In summary, NOTCH acquires a tumour suppressive role through the alteration of the canonical signalling pathway in neuroendocrine lung cancers. It could be interesting to explore the possible therapeutic strategies restoring the expression of NOTCH-mutated components in SCLC, or targeting the DDL3 in order to direct cytotoxic drugs.

5.3. Role of NOTCH in Neuroendocrine Gastro-Entero-Pancreatic Neuroendocrine Neoplasms (GEP-NENs)

The gastrointestinal (GI) tract and the pancreas are two of the most common sites of origin for NENs. Tumours arising from these organs are named gastro-entero-pancreatic NENs (GEP-NENs) and they represent almost the 65% of all NENs. Previously GEP-NENs were considered as a unique group of tumours, however, currently, many studies have highlighted the biological and molecular differences between pancreatic and GI NENs, as well as between the GI NENs originating from different organs of the GI tract [11,15,16,18]. Wang et al. have confirmed this heterogeneity in their study related to the implication of the NOTCH signalling pathway [105]. They demonstrated a uniform immune-histochemical expression of NOTCH1 and HES1 in well-differentiated rectal NENs—found to be, respectively, 100% and 64%—whereas only 34% and 10% of well-differentiated pancreatic NENs were positive for NOTCH1 and HES1 at immunohistochemistry, and all ileal NENs were negative to both, suggesting a possible different role of NOTCH1 in the pathogenesis of these cancers. [105].

The majority of the available studies have evaluated the role of NOTCH signalling in pancreatic NENs, thus there is a lack of knowledge on the role of NOTCH signalling in the other GEP-NENs.

In the pancreas, endocrine and exocrine cells move from a common pool of multipotent progenitors into a differentiated state, co-ordinately regulated by different mechanisms, forming together a complete and functional adult organ. After the initial developmental phase, the epithelium starts to spread pancreatic progenitor cells into different compartments: acinar cells migrated into the tips, and ductal and endocrine cells into the trunk. Endocrine cells leave the adjacent epithelia by delamination, assembling into islets of Langerhans. During the differentiation process, the mechanism of differentiation is not synchronous, and it is controlled by several regulatory agents, such as the NOTCH receptor that has an important role in the early developmental embryologic phase, as well as in adult plasticity.

In aggressive tumours of the pancreas-like pancreatic ductal adenocarcinomas (PDAC), the tumour is believed to derive from a pancreatic intraperitoneal neoplasia (PanIN). In these cases, Notch plays a dual role in the tumour initiation and development—NOTCH works as a tumour suppressor in PanIN lesions [106] and later on it has an oncogenic role in PDAC [107]. Furthermore, these studies indicate not only this dual role of the NOTCH pathway in tumorigenesis, but also the implication of several pathway components, revealing a complex fine-tuning regulation of the NOTCH pathway.

Moreover, histo-pathological studies have shown that NOTCH1 is absent or poorly-expressed in well-differentiated pancreatic neuroendocrine tumours (pNET) [8,105]. However, in MiNEN (mixed neuroendocrine/non neuroendocrine neoplasm), the expression of NOTCH1 and Hes1 is reduced or absent in the neuroendocrine cells, but both NOTCH1 and Hes1 are present in the adenomatous component [84], potentially indicating a possible role of NOTCH as a tumour suppressor gene. Further studies are needed to characterise the molecular mechanisms implicated in neuroendocrine tumorigenesis and for the understanding of the functional differences observed within pancreatic tumours.

In ileal NENs, the low or absent expression of NOTCH and HES1 has led to hypnotize a possible tumour suppressor role of the NOTCH canonical signalling cascade [105]. As confirmation of this hypothesis, Maggi et al. [108] demonstrated that Retinoblastoma-binding protein 2 (RBP2), a key component of the NOTCH repressor complex, is upregulated in gastrointestinal NENs and in liver metastases. Nonetheless, further studies are needed to confirm the role of NOTCH signalling in GI-NENs and to drive an effective therapeutic strategy modulating the NOTCH pathway in these tumours.

5.4. Role of NOTCH in Medullary Thyroid Cancer

Medullary thyroid cancer (MTC) is a neuroendocrine tumour that emerges from parafollicular C-cells of the thyroid gland. In MTC, the proliferation of neuroendocrine cells and tumour growth process appears to be regulated by a common pathway. A major role is played by the ASCL1 transcription factor, highly expressed in MTC, that is involved in supporting cell proliferation and embryologic precursor survival, as well as inhibiting apoptosis [109].

The canonical NOTCH signalling cascade directly reduces the expression of ASCL1, with an anti-proliferative effect. A decrease in NOTCH1 and NOTCH3 expression has been documented in MTC [81,110]. The activation of doxycycline-inducible NOTCH1 and NOTCH3 in TT cells, through treatment with increased doses of doxycycline, has demonstrated a dose-dependent increase in NOTCH1, NOTCH3 and HES1 protein, a decrease in ASCL1 levels and ultimately a reduction in tumour growth in vitro and in vivo. A decrease in the production of chromogranin A neuropeptides and specific neuron enolase (NSE), two of the main MTC biomarkers, has been also documented [81,110].

The same results were obtained by the pharmacological NOTCH3 induction, with the activating compounds AB3 suggesting NOTCH3 as a potential target for MTC treatment [111].

Moreover, the dedifferentiation process, typical of thyroid oncogenesis, seems to be correlated with the loss of NOTCH3 expression, whereas the doxycycline-induced NOTCH3 activation restores the differentiated phenotype and has an antiproliferative effect in thyroid cancer cell lines (TT, FTC) [81,111].

5.5. Role of NOTCH in Malignant Castration-Resistant Prostatic Cells

Prostatic small-cell carcinoma, originating from neuroendocrine diffuse cells in the prostate, is a rare neoplasia with a lack of understanding in tumour development and progression, as well as in useful prognostic factors and genetic biomarkers. More often, in prostatic cancer (PCa), prostatic cells lose the maintenance of tissue identity and by a lineage-plasticity manner transdifferentiate in the neuroendocrine phenotype following androgen deprivation therapy.

The neuroendocrine cells promote hormone-resistance, secreting peptides that can stimulate androgen-dependent growth, and reducing apoptosis. Neuroendocrine cells do not express androgenic receptors, as they are not sensitive to the therapy of androgenic deprivation and have poor sensitivity to standard chemotherapeutic agents. Interestingly, this fact seems to be related with tumour plasticity for the epithelial mesenchymal transition (EMT) process and with the alteration of the signalling pathway regulators involved in cellular proliferation and differentiation.

Currently, there are ongoing studies aimed to explore the role of NOTCH in malignant castration-resistant prostatic cancer models. Preliminary investigations revealed that hypoxia, which is linked to PCa progression, induces neuroendocrine differentiation (NED) in androgen-sensitive prostate cancer cells (LNCaP) through the downregulation of NOTCH1 and NOTCH2 mRNA and protein expression with the subsequent reduction of HES1 transcription [112]. In addition, gene profiling of castration-resistant neuroendocrine prostate cancer (NEPC) samples showed that some Notch-related genes (DLL3, DLL4, HES6, DTX1 and JAG2) are up-regulated, and others (NOTCH2 and 4) are considerably down-regulated. This fact suggests a dual role of NOTCH signalling in NEPC. Of note, in the same study, DLL3 protein expression was evaluated and it was found to be present in 76.6% of castration-resistant NEPC, but only in the 12.5% of castration-resistant prostate adenocarcinomas. This fact proposes DLL3 as a possible biomarker of NED and a potential therapeutic target for the treatment of DLL3-positive metastatic prostate cancer [113].

6. Therapeutic Approach Targeting NOTCH in NENs

A pharmacological modulation of the NOTCH pathway is an interesting concept to pursue for neuroendocrine tumour treatment. Overall, there are several approaches to modulate NOTCH signalling that are in different stages of development in cancer treatment. Among them, there are NOTCH-inhibiting and NOTCH-activating strategies.

The evidence gathered to date suggests that NOTCH is a tumour suppressor in NENs; however, a putative pro-oncogenic role of NOTCH signalling has been suggested for the non-neuroendocrine components of NENs and has been linked with NEN heterogeneity [73]. Thus, preliminary studies have evaluated the efficacy of both NOTCH-activating and NOTCH-inhibiting strategies.

In particular, with regard to the NOTCH-activating compounds, histone deacetylase inhibitors and valproic acid (VA) showed an in vitro antineoplastic effect in neuroendocrine cell lines (gastrointestinal carcinoid, broncopulmonary carcinoid and in human medullary thyroid cancer cell lines), inducing NOTCH1 mRNA expression through activator protein (AP) transcription factor binding [114]. In addition, in neuroendocrine cells, VA was shown to stimulate the expression of somatostatin receptor type 2 (SSTR2) that is largely targeted in neuroendocrine anticancer therapy [115]. This suggests a potential role of VA in these tumours to get a sensitization to SSTR2-targeted therapy. The efficacy of VA has also been tested in a phase II clinical trial, in which patients with G1/G2 neuroendocrine tumours treated with VA achieved relative good tumour control [116]. However, it remains unclear if the efficacy of VA in NENs is specifically related to the activation of NOTCH signalling, or if it is also related to the direct or indirect regulation of other pathways.

Therefore, a more specific targeted therapy for NOTCH signalling activation is needed. To date, there are few compounds that specifically activate NOTCH signalling and are in a very early stage of development. One example is a NOTCH3-specific antibody that binds to the NRR, causing conformational changes in the NOTCH receptor that renders S2 cleavage sites accessible to ADAMs. This antibody has been preliminary tested in 293T cells as "proof of principle" of NOTCH3 activation [117]. Thus, further studies are warranted.

The lack of big data on NOTCH-activating compounds is mainly due to the fact that in the majority of cancers, NOTCH acts as an oncogene, and, consequently, the efforts of the scientific community have been focused on the development of NOTCH-inhibiting strategies. These inhibiting strategies have been tested also in NEN treatment, studied alone or in combination with chemotherapy. The rationale behind the use of NOTCH-inhibiting drugs in NEN is mainly based on the possibility of keeping under control the non-neuroendocrine component of the tumour, preventing the neuroendocrine-to-non-neuroendocrine cell fate switch. The addition of chemotherapy is aimed to kill the neuroendocrine cells that are chemosensitive. In particular, tarextumab, a Notch2/Notch3 antagonist, has been tested alone and in combination with chemotherapy in vivo SCLC models [77], and in patients with SCLC [118]. Although in the pre-clinical models (SCLC allografts and patient-derived xenograft) the combination of tarextumab with carboplatin and irinotecan achieved a better tumour inhibition than chemotherapy or tarextumab alone [77], the clinical trial was unsuccessful, not meeting the primary endpoint of progression free survival (PFS) [118]. In an explorative clinical phase I trial, the γ-secretase NOTCH inhibitor RO4929097 was tested in solid malignancies, and within this trial a patient affected by colorectal cancer with neuroendocrine feature achieved a partial response [119].

Therefore, the results obtained with the NOTCH-inhibiting treatment in NENs are discordant. Future research should be aimed to select the patients, in relation to the characteristics of the tumour and the optimal timing within the course of the disease, in which the administration of NOTCH inhibitors could be most beneficial to reduce heterogeneity.

Lastly, a different approach that is neither activating nor inhibiting of NOTCH pathway, but instead targets the DLL3 NOTCH ligand, is the one behind the treatment with Rova-T. Rova-T is an antibody-drug conjugate recently tested in SCLC and neuroendocrine prostate cancer (NEPC). It is composed of a humanized monoclonal antibody directed against DLL3 and a cytotoxic payload (tesirine), and uses the DLL3 to direct the cytotoxic drug into the tumour cells. Rova-T has been tested in the phase II TRINITY trial and in the phase III TAHOE trial as third- and second-line, respectively, in patients with DLL3-positive SCLC [120,121], following the promising results of pre-clinical studies and a phase I trial [122]. In the TRINITY trial, the best overall response rate achieved with Rova-T treatment was 29% (95% confidence interval (CI), 22–36) and 16% (95% CI, 11–22) according to the investigator and the independent review committee assessment, respectively. The median overall survival was 5.6 months (95% CI, 4.9–6.8) in the overall enrolled population, while it was 6.7 in the DLL3-high ($\geq$75% tumour cells positive for DLL3 by immunohistochemistry) patients.

Unfortunately, the enrolment in the TAHOE trial was stopped because of the shorter overall survival (OS) reported in the Rova-T arm compared with the control arm (topotecan treatment).

However, despite these unfavourable results, Rova-T is currently under investigation in the phase III MERU trial (NCT03033511), which compares Rova-T to placebo as maintenance therapy after platinum-based chemotherapy in patients with extensive-stage SCLC. In addition, phase I studies are also evaluating Rova-T in combination with first-line chemotherapy (cisplatin/etoposide), nivolumab and nivolumab plus ipilimumab in NSLC. Rova-T is also under investigation as treatment for patients with NEPC (NCT02709889), following the excellent pre-clinical results [123]. The results of these trials are strongly awaited.

The evidence gathered to date is not strong enough to draw a general conclusion on the optimal NOTCH modulatory strategy to be pursued for NEN treatment. However, it seems that NOTCH inhibition could be needed to reduce tumour heterogeneity within the NENs; however, once the neuroendocrine phenotype is established, NOTCH activation should be targeted. A limitation of the NOTCH-activating approach is the possible off-target oncogenic effect on other tissues that could result in higher damage to the patient. Thus, strategies to ensure a high target specificity are required. Two possible attractive solutions to this problem could be the development of bi-specific antibodies and/or functionalized nanoparticles carrying a NOTCH activator [124,125]. In the first approach, antibodies are generated to bind to two different antigens, with one usually being the therapeutic target and the other being a specific marker of the tumour to treat. This conformation ensures specific therapeutic activity at the tumour side, ultimately reducing the off-target effect. For the NEN treatment, a possible bi-specific antibody could target epidermal growth factor receptor (EGFR) with an antagonistic effect and NOTCH with an activating effect. A similar approach has already been successfully tested in other cancers, but instead using an EGFR/NOTCH antagonist antibody [126]. In the second approach, nanoparticles are functionalized with different peptides to efficiently deliver the targeted drug that is loaded into the nanoparticle itself. An attractive hypothesis for the treatment of somatostatin receptor positive NEN treatment would be functionalize the nanoparticle-carrying NOTCH activator with tumour-inhibiting somatostatin analogues. However, this represents a preliminary hypothesis that must first be tested.

7. Conclusions

Although several studies have been conducted with the aim of identifying genetic mutations involved in the genesis of neuroendocrine tumours, none of them have shown a substantial mutational percentage in the samples analysed, revealing a low-abundance of consistent mutations in G1/G2 neoplasms compared with other malignancies. Moreover, the modern sequencing technologies highlighted heterogeneity of mutations depending on the tumour anatomic origin.

For these reasons, there are still many unknowns in the genomic characterization of NETs in comparison with other neoplasia, with the majority of the data covering predominantly pancreatic, lung and small-intestine NET.

Therefore, multi-centre collaborations, international databases, biological banks and genome-wide profiling overture should be pursued.

The NOTCH pathway has recently emerged as key factor in NEN development and progression, and it seems to play an important role in generating NEN intra-tumour heterogeneity. NOTCH signalling mainly has a tumour-suppressive role in NENs, justifying the use of NOTCH-activating strategies for their treatment. However, a proto-oncogenic role has been suggested in the non-neuroendocrine components of NENs that generates a fertile microenvironment for the development of neuroendocrine tumours, thus also the NOTCH-inhibiting approach has been considered in NEN treatment.

To date, both NOTCH-activating and NOTCH-inhibiting approaches are still at a very early phase of development as therapy for NENs, whereas more advanced but debatable results have been achieved with Rova-T treatment.

In conclusion, the role of NOTCH as a therapeutic target in NENs, as well as the currently available therapeutic strategies for targeting this pathway, have to be further investigated and developed. In particular, future research should be aimed at elucidating the possible specific targets within the NOTCH pathway susceptible to pharmacological regulation, and to identify specific tumour markers that could be used to deliver NOTCH-modulator agents to the tumour cells, as well as unveil specific biomarkers that could better stratify the group of patients that could benefit from a NOTCH-activating and/or inhibiting therapy.

Author Contributions: S.T., M.L.T. and C.v.A. have contributed to the conceptualization; C.v.A., E.L.-J., M.C. have equally contributed to the search of the literature and writing of the original draft of this manuscript; C.v.A., E.L.-J., A.D.M., F.T., A.O., G.N., M.L.T. and S.T. have reviewed and edited the final version of the manuscript; A.O. and C.v.A. have elaborated the figures; S.T. supervised the team. All authors read and approved the final manuscript.

Acknowledgments: We thank the close collaboration of the no-profit organization Lega Italiana Per La Lotta Contro i Tumori (LILT) of Naples, and Alessandra Trocino, librarian at the Library of Istituto Nazionale Tumori Fondazione 'G Pascale', Naples, Italy, for her excellent bibliographic service and assistance.

Conflicts of Interest: The authors declare no conflict of interest.

References

1. Merrell, A.J.; Stanger, B.Z. Adult cell plasticity in vivo: De-differentiation and transdifferentiation are back in style. *Nat. Rev. Mol. Cell Biol.* **2016**, *17*, 413–425. [CrossRef] [PubMed]
2. Artavanis-Tsakonas, S.; Rand, M.D.; Lake, R.J. Notch signaling: Cell fate control and signal integration in development. *Science* **1999**, *284*, 770–776. [CrossRef] [PubMed]
3. Shih, H.P.; Kopp, J.L.; Sandhu, M.; Dubois, C.L.; Seymour, P.A.; Grapin-Botton, A.; Sander, M. A Notch-dependent molecular circuitry initiates pancreatic endocrine and ductal cell differentiation. *Development* **2012**, *139*, 2488–2499. [CrossRef] [PubMed]
4. Patel, P.; Galoian, K. Molecular challenges of neuroendocrine tumors. *Oncol. Lett.* **2018**, *15*, 2715–2725. [CrossRef] [PubMed]
5. Chikara, S.; Reindl, K.M. NOTCH signaling: A hero or villain in the war against cancer? *Transl. Lung Cancer Res.* **2013**, *2*, 449–451. [CrossRef] [PubMed]
6. Carter, Y.; Jaskula-Sztul, R.; Chen, H.; Mazeh, H. Signaling pathways as specific pharmacologic targets for neuroendocrine tumor therapy: RET, PI3K, MEK, growth factors, and NOTCH. *Neuroendocrinology* **2013**, *97*, 57–66. [CrossRef]
7. Hassan, W.A.; Yoshida, R.; Kudoh, S.; Hasegawa, K.; Niimori-Kita, K.; Ito, T. Notch1 controls cell invasion and metastasis in small cell lung carcinoma cell lines. *Lung Cancer* **2014**, *86*, 304–310. [CrossRef]
8. Krausch, M.; Kroepil, F.; Lehwald, N.; Lachenmayer, A.; Schott, M.; Anlauf, M.; Cupisti, K.; Knoefel, W.T.; Raffel, A. NOTCH 1 tumor expression is lacking in highly proliferative pancreatic neuroendocrine tumors. *Endocrine* **2013**, *44*, 182–186. [CrossRef]
9. Kunnimalaiyaan, M.; Chen, H. Tumor suppressor role of notch-1 signaling in neuroendocrine tumors. *Oncologist* **2007**, *12*, 535–542. [CrossRef]
10. Kunnimalaiyaan, M.; Yan, S.; Wong, F.; Zhang, Y.W.; Chen, H. Hairy enhancer of split-1 (HES-1), a Notch1 effector, inhibits the growth of carcinoid tumor cells. *Surgery* **2005**, *138*, 1137–1142. [CrossRef]
11. Banck, M.S.; Kanwar, R.; Kulkarni, A.A.; Boora, G.K.; Metge, F.; Kipp, B.R.; Zhang, L.; Thorland, E.C.; Minn, K.T.; Tentu, R.; et al. The genomic landscape of small intestine neuroendocrine tumors. *J. Clin. Investig.* **2013**, *123*, 2502–2508. [CrossRef] [PubMed]
12. Pelosi, G.; Bianchi, F.; Hofman, P.; Pattini, L.; Ströbel, P.; Calabrese, F.; Naheed, S.; Holden, C.; Cave, J.; Bohnenberger, H.; et al. Recent advances in the molecular landscape of lung neuroendocrine tumors. *Expert Rev. Mol. Diagn.* **2019**, *19*, 281–297. [CrossRef] [PubMed]
13. Wong, H.L.; Yang, K.C.; Shen, Y.; Zhao, E.Y.; Loree, J.M.; Kennecke, H.F.; Kalloger, S.E.; Karasinska, J.M.; Lim, H.J.; Mungall, A.J.; et al. Molecular characterization of metastatic pancreatic neuroendocrine tumors (PNETs) using whole-genome and transcriptome sequencing. *Cold Spring Harb. Mol. Case Stud.* **2018**, *4*. [CrossRef] [PubMed]
14. Rickman, D.S.; Beltran, H.; Demichelis, F.; Rubin, M.A. Biology and evolution of poorly differentiated neuroendocrine tumors. *Nat. Med.* **2017**, *23*, 664–673. [CrossRef] [PubMed]

15. Jiao, Y.; Shi, C.; Edil, B.H.; De Wilde, R.F.; Klimstra, D.S.; Maitra, A.; Schulick, R.D.; Tang, L.H.; Wolfgang, C.L.; Choti, M.A.; et al. DAXX/ATRX, MEN1 and mTOR pathway genes are frequently altered in pancreatic neuroendocrine tumors. *Science* **2011**, *331*, 1199–1203. [CrossRef] [PubMed]
16. Scarpa, A.; Initiative, A.P.C.G.; Chang, D.K.; Nones, K.; Corbo, V.; Patch, A.M.; Bailey, P.; Lawlor, R.T.; Johns, A.L.; Miller, D.K.; et al. Whole-genome landscape of pancreatic neuroendocrine tumours. *Nature* **2017**, *543*, 65–71. [CrossRef] [PubMed]
17. Jensen, R.T.; Berna, M.J.; Bingham, D.B.; Norton, J.A. Inherited pancreatic endocrine tumor syndromes: Advances in molecular pathogenesis, diagnosis, management and controversies. *Cancer* **2008**, *113*, 1807–1843. [CrossRef] [PubMed]
18. Francis, J.M.; Kiezun, A.; Ramos, A.H.; Serra, S.; Pedamallu, C.S.; Qian, Z.R.; Banck, M.S.; Kanwar, R.; Kulkarni, A.A.; Karpathakis, A.; et al. Somatic mutation of CDKN1B in small intestine neuroendocrine tumors. *Nat. Genet.* **2013**, *45*, 1483–1486. [CrossRef]
19. Singhi, A.D.; Liu, T.C.; Roncaioli, J.L.; Cao, D.; Zeh, H.J.; Zureikat, A.H.; Tsung, A.; Marsh, J.W.; Lee, K.K.; Hogg, M.E.; et al. Alternative lengthening of telomeres and loss of DAXX/ATRX expression predicts metastatic disease and poor survival in patients with pancreatic neuroendocrine tumors. *Clin. Cancer Res.* **2017**, *23*, 600–609. [CrossRef] [PubMed]
20. Vijayvergia, N.; Boland, P.M.; Handorf, E.; Gustafson, K.S.; Gong, Y.; Cooper, H.S.; Sheriff, F.; Astsaturov, I.; Cohen, S.J.; Engstrom, P.F. Molecular profiling of neuroendocrine malignancies to identify prognostic and therapeutic markers: A Fox Chase Cancer Center Pilot Study. *Br. J. Cancer* **2016**, *115*, 564–570. [CrossRef] [PubMed]
21. Öberg, K. The Genetics of neuroendocrine tumors. *Semin. Oncol.* **2013**, *40*, 37–44. [CrossRef] [PubMed]
22. Marx, S.J. Recent topics around multiple endocrine neoplasia type. *J. Clin. Endocrinol. Metab.* **2018**, *103*, 1296–1301. [CrossRef] [PubMed]
23. Frost, M.; Lines, K.E.; Thakker, R.V. Current and emerging therapies for PNETs in patients with or without MEN1. *Nat. Rev. Endocrinol.* **2018**, *14*, 216–227. [CrossRef] [PubMed]
24. Pepe, S.; Korbonits, M.; Iacovazzo, D. Germline and mosaic mutations causing pituitary tumours: Genetic and molecular aspects. *J. Endocrinol.* **2019**, *240*, R21–R45. [CrossRef] [PubMed]
25. Khatami, F.; Tavangar, S.M. Multiple endocrine neoplasia syndromes from genetic and epigenetic Perspectives. *Biomark. Insights* **2018**, *13*. [CrossRef]
26. Ren, F.; Xu, H.W.; Hu, Y.; Yan, S.H.; Wang, F.; Su, B.W.; Zhao, Q. Expression and subcellular localization of menin in human cancer cells. *Exp. Ther. Med.* **2012**, *3*, 1087–1091. [CrossRef]
27. Petr, E.J.; Else, T. Genetic predisposition to endocrine tumors: Diagnosis, surveillance and challenges in care. *Semin. Oncol.* **2016**, *43*, 582–590. [CrossRef]
28. Plaza-Menacho, I. Structure and function of RET in multiple endocrine neoplasia type 2. *Endocr. Relat. Cancer* **2018**, *25*, T79–T90. [CrossRef]
29. Wells, S.A.; Pacini, F.; Robinson, B.G.; Santoro, M. Multiple Endocrine Neoplasia Type 2 and Familial Medullary Thyroid Carcinoma: An Update. *J. Clin. Endocrinol. Metab.* **2013**, *98*, 3149–3164. [CrossRef]
30. Pellegata, N.S.; Quintanilla-Martinez, L.; Siggelkow, H.; Samson, E.; Bink, K.; Höfler, H.; Fend, F.; Graw, J.; Atkinson, M.J. Germ-line mutations in p27Kip1 cause a multiple endocrine neoplasia syndrome in rats and humans. *Proc. Natl. Acad. Sci. USA* **2006**, *103*, 15558–15563. [CrossRef]
31. Varshney, N.; Kebede, A.A.; Owusu-Dapaah, H.; Lather, J.; Kaushik, M.; Bhullar, J.S. A review of von hippel-lindau syndrome. *J. Kidney Cancer VHL* **2017**, *4*, 20–29. [CrossRef] [PubMed]
32. López-Jiménez, E.; Gómez-López, G.; Leandro-García, L.J.; Muñoz, I.; Schiavi, F.; Montero-Conde, C.; De Cubas, A.A.; Ramires, R.; Landa, I.; Leskela, S.; et al. Research resource: transcriptional profiling reveals different pseudohypoxic signatures in SDHB and VHL-Related pheochromocytomas. *Mol. Endocrinol.* **2010**, *24*, 2382–2391. [CrossRef] [PubMed]
33. Dahia, P.L.; Ross, K.N.; Wright, M.E.; Hayashida, C.Y.; Santagata, S.; Barontini, M.; Kung, A.L.; Sanso, G.; Powers, J.F.; Tischler, A.S.; et al. A HIF1alpha regulatory loop links hypoxia and mitochondrial signals in pheochromocytomas. *PLoS Genet.* **2005**, *1*, 72–80. [CrossRef] [PubMed]
34. Maeda, Y.; Suzuki, T.; Pan, X.; Chen, G.; Pan, S.; Bartman, T.; Whitsett, J.A. CUL2 Is Required for the activity of hypoxia-inducible factor and vasculogenesis. *J. Boil. Chem.* **2008**, *283*, 16084–16092. [CrossRef] [PubMed]

35. Miyauchi, Y.; Kato, M.; Tokunaga, F.; Iwai, K. The COP9/signalosome increases the efficiency of von hippel-lindau protein ubiquitin ligase-mediated hypoxia-inducible factor-ubiquitination. *J. Boil. Chem.* **2008**, *283*, 16622–16631. [CrossRef] [PubMed]
36. Ku, Y.H.; Ahn, C.H.; Jung, C.H.; Lee, J.E.; Kim, L.K.; Kwak, S.H.; Jung, H.S.; Park, K.S.; Cho, Y.M. A novel mutation in the von hippel-lindau tumor suppressor gene identified in a patient presenting with gestational diabetes mellitus. *Endocrinol. Metab.* **2013**, *28*, 320–325. [CrossRef] [PubMed]
37. Lodish, M.B.; Stratakis, C.A. Endocrine tumours in neurofibromatosis type 1, tuberous sclerosis and related syndromes. *Best Pract. Res. Clin. Endocrinol. Metab.* **2010**, *24*, 439–449. [CrossRef] [PubMed]
38. De Luca, A.; Bottillo, I.; Dasdia, M.C.; Morella, A.; Lanari, V.; Bernardini, L.; Divona, L.; Giustini, S.; Sinibaldi, L.; Novelli, A.; et al. Deletions of NF1 gene and exons detected by multiplex ligation-dependent probe amplification. *J. Med. Genet.* **2007**, *44*, 800–808. [CrossRef] [PubMed]
39. Rachdi, L.; Balcazar, N.; Osorio-Duque, F.; Elghazi, L.; Weiss, A.; Gould, A.; Chang-Chen, K.J.; Gambello, M.J.; Bernal-Mizrachi, E. Disruption of Tsc2 in pancreatic beta cells induces beta cell mass expansion and improved glucose tolerance in a TORC1-dependent manner. *Proc. Natl. Acad. Sci. USA* **2008**, *105*, 9250–9255. [CrossRef] [PubMed]
40. Willenberg, H.; Lehwald, N.; Hafner, D.; Knoefel, W.T.; Krausch, M.; Raffel, A.; Anlauf, M.; Schott, M.; Cupisti, K.; Eisenberger, C.F. Loss of PTEN expression in neuroendocrine pancreatic tumors. *Horm. Metab. Res.* **2011**, *43*, 865–871.
41. Lefebvre, M.; Foulkes, W.D. Pheochromocytoma and paraganglioma syndromes: Genetics and management update. *Curr. Oncol.* **2014**, *21*, e8–e17. [CrossRef] [PubMed]
42. Ricketts, C.J.; Forman, J.R.; Rattenberry, E.; Bradshaw, N.; Lalloo, F.; Izatt, L.; Cole, T.R.; Armstrong, R.; Kumar, V.K.; Morrison, P.J.; et al. Tumor risks and genotype-phenotype-proteotype analysis in 358 patients with germline mutations in SDHB and SDHD. *Hum. Mutat.* **2010**, *31*, 41–51. [CrossRef] [PubMed]
43. Guzy, R.D.; Sharma, B.; Bell, E.; Chandel, N.S.; Schumacker, P.T. Loss of the SdhB, but Not the SdhA, subunit of complex II triggers reactive oxygen species-dependent hypoxia-inducible factor activation and tumorigenesis. *Mol. Cell Biol.* **2008**, *28*, 718–731. [CrossRef] [PubMed]
44. Burnichon, N.; Brière, J.J.; Libé, R.; Vescovo, L.; Rivière, J.; Tissier, F.; Jouanno, E.; Jeunemaitre, X.; Bénit, P.; Tzagoloff, A.; et al. SDHA is a tumor suppressor gene causing paraganglioma. *Hum. Mol. Genet.* **2010**, *19*, 3011–3020. [CrossRef] [PubMed]
45. Gimenez-Roqueplo, A.P.; Favier, J.; Rustin, P.; Rieubland, C.; Crespin, M.; Nau, V.; Khau Van Kien, P.; Corvol, P.; Plouin, P.F.; Jeunemaitre, X.; et al. Mutations in the SDHB gene are associated with extra-adrenal and/or malignant phaeochromocytomas. *Cancer Res.* **2003**, *63*, 5615–5621.
46. Hao, H.X.; Khalimonchuk, O.; Schraders, M.; Dephoure, N.; Bayley, J.P.; Kunst, H.; Devilee, P.; Cremers, C.W.; Schiffman, J.D.; Bentz, B.G.; et al. SDH5, a gene required for flavination of succinate dehydrogenase, is mutated in paraganglioma. *Science* **2009**, *325*, 1139–1142. [CrossRef] [PubMed]
47. Astuti, D.; Latif, F.; Dallol, A.; Dahia, P.L.; Douglas, F.; George, E.; Sköldberg, F.; Husebye, E.S.; Eng, C.; Maher, E.R.; et al. Gene mutations in the succinate dehydrogenase subunit SDHB cause susceptibility to familial pheochromocytoma and to familial paraganglioma. *Am. J. Hum. Genet.* **2001**, *69*, 49–54. [CrossRef]
48. Niemann, S.; Müller, U. Mutations in SDHC cause autosomal dominant paraganglioma, type 3. *Nat. Genet.* **2000**, *26*, 268–270. [CrossRef]
49. Niemann, S.; Müller, U.; Engelhardt, D.; Lohse, P. Autosomal dominant malignant and catecholamine-producing paraganglioma caused by a splice donor site mutation in SDHC. *Hum. Genet.* **2003**, *113*, 92–94.
50. Baysal, B.E. Mutations in SDHD, a mitochondrial complex II gene, in hereditary paraganglioma. *Science* **2000**, *287*, 848–851. [CrossRef]
51. Ugarte-Camara, M.; Fernandez-Prado, R.; Lorda, I.; Rosselló, G.; Gonzalez-Enguita, C.; Cannata-Ortiz, P.; Ortiz, A. Positive/retained SDHB immunostaining in renal cell carcinomas associated to germline SDHB-deficiency: Case report. *Diagn. Pathol.* **2019**, *14*, 42. [CrossRef] [PubMed]
52. Eijkelenkamp, K.; Osinga, T.E.; Links, T.P.; Horst-Schrivers, A.N.; Van Der Horst-Schrivers, A.N. Clinical implications of the oncometabolite succinate in SDHx-mutation carriers. *Clin. Genet.* **2019**. [CrossRef] [PubMed]
53. Crona, J.; Skogseid, B. GEP—NETS UPDATE: Genetics of neuroendocrine tumors. *Eur. J. Endocrinol.* **2016**, *174*, R275–R290. [CrossRef] [PubMed]

54. Yachida, S.; Vakiani, E.; White, C.M.; Zhong, Y.; Saunders, T.; Morgan, R.; De Wilde, R.F.; Maitra, A.; Hicks, J.; DeMarzo, A.M.; et al. Small cell and large cell neuroendocrine carcinomas of the pancreas are genetically similar and distinct from well-differentiated pancreatic neuroendocrine tumors. *Am. J. Surg. Pathol.* **2012**, *36*, 173–184. [CrossRef] [PubMed]
55. Basturk, O.; Yang, Z.; Tang, L.H.; Hruban, R.H.; Adsay, N.V.; McCall, C.M.; Krasinskas, A.M.; Jang, K.T.; Frankel, W.L.; Balci, S.; et al. The high grade (Who G3) pancreatic neuroendocrine tumor category is morphologically and biologically heterogeneous and includes both well differentiated and poorly differentiated neoplasms. *Am. J. Surg. Pathol.* **2015**, *39*, 683–690. [CrossRef]
56. Scarpa, A.; Mantovani, W.; Capelli, P.; Beghelli, S.; Boninsegna, L.; Bettini, R.; Panzuto, F.; Pederzoli, P.; Fave, G.D.; Falconi, M. Pancreatic endocrine tumors: Improved TNM staging and histopathological grading permit a clinically efficient prognostic stratification of patients. *Mod. Pathol.* **2010**, *23*, 824–833. [CrossRef]
57. Vélayoudom-Céphise, F.L.; Duvillard, P.; Foucan, L.; Hadoux, J.; Chougnet, C.N.; Leboulleux, S.; Malka, D.; Guigay, J.; Goere, D.; Debaere, T.; et al. Are G3 ENETS neuroendocrine neoplasms heterogeneous? *Endocr. Relat. Cancer* **2013**, *20*, 649–657. [CrossRef]
58. George, J.; Lim, J.S.; Jang, S.J.; Cun, Y.; Ozretić, L.; Kong, G.; Leenders, F.; Lü, X.; Fernandez-Cuesta, L.; Bosco, G.; et al. Comprehensive genomic profiles of small cell lung cancer. *Nature* **2015**, *524*, 47–53. [CrossRef]
59. Makuuchi, R.; Terashima, M.; Kusuhara, M.; Nakajima, T.; Serizawa, M.; Hatakeyama, K.; Ohshima, K.; Urakami, K.; Yamaguchi, K. Comprehensive analysis of gene mutation and expression profiles in neuroendocrine carcinomas of the stomach. *Biomed. Res.* **2017**, *38*, 19–27. [CrossRef]
60. Takizawa, N.; Ohishi, Y.; Hirahashi, M.; Takahashi, S.; Nakamura, K.; Tanaka, M.; Oki, E.; Takayanagi, R.; Oda, Y. Molecular characteristics of colorectal neuroendocrine carcinoma; similarities with adenocarcinoma rather than neuroendocrine tumor. *Hum. Pathol.* **2015**, *46*, 1890–1900. [CrossRef]
61. Ali, A.S.; Grönberg, M.; Federspiel, B.; Scoazec, J.Y.; Hjortland, G.O.; Grønbæk, H.; Ladekarl, M.; Langer, S.W.; Welin, S.; Vestermark, L.W.; et al. Expression of p53 protein in high-grade gastroenteropancreatic neuroendocrine carcinoma. *PLoS ONE* **2017**, *12*, e0187667. [CrossRef] [PubMed]
62. Sahnane, N.; Furlan, D.; Monti, M.; Romualdi, C.; Vanoli, A.; Vicari, E.; Solcia, E.; Capella, C.; Sessa, F.; La Rosa, S. Microsatellite unstable gastrointestinal neuroendocrine carcinomas: A new clinicopathologic entity. *Endocr. Relat. Cancer* **2015**, *22*, 35–45. [CrossRef] [PubMed]
63. Olevian, D.C.; Nikiforovag, M.N.; Chiosea, S.; Sun, W.; Bahary, N.; Kuan, S.F.; Pai, R.K. Colorectal poorly differentiated neuroendocrine carcinomas frequently exhibit BRAF mutations and are associated with poor overall survival. *Hum. Pathol.* **2016**, *49*, 124–134. [CrossRef] [PubMed]
64. Jesinghaus, M.; Konukiewitz, B.; Keller, G.; Kloor, M.; Steiger, K.; Reiche, M.; Penzel, R.; Endris, V.; Arsenic, R.; Hermann, G.; et al. Colorectal mixed adenoneuroendocrine carcinomas and neuroendocrine carcinomas are genetically closely related to colorectal adenocarcinomas. *Mod. Pathol.* **2017**, *30*, 610–619. [CrossRef] [PubMed]
65. Hijioka, S.; Hosoda, W.; Mizuno, N.; Hara, K.; Imaoka, H.; Bhatia, V.; Mekky, M.A.; Tajika, M.; Tanaka, T.; Ishihara, M.; et al. Does the WHO 2010 classification of pancreatic neuroendocrine neoplasms accurately characterize pancreatic neuroendocrine carcinomas? *J. Gastroenterol.* **2015**, *50*, 564–572. [CrossRef] [PubMed]
66. Woischke, C.; Schaaf, C.W.; Yang, H.M.; Vieth, M.; Veits, L.; Geddert, H.; Märkl, B.; Stömmer, P.; Schaeffer, D.F.; Frölich, M.; et al. In-depth mutational analyses of colorectal neuroendocrine carcinomas with adenoma or adenocarcinoma components. *Mod. Pathol.* **2017**, *30*, 95–103. [CrossRef] [PubMed]
67. Karkouche, R.; Bachet, J.B.; Sandrini, J.; Mitry, E.; Penna, C.; Côté, J.F.; Blons, H.; Penault-Llorca, F.; Rougier, P.; André, J.P.S.; et al. Colorectal neuroendocrine carcinomas and adenocarcinomas share oncogenic pathways. A clinico-pathologic study of 12 cases. *Eur. J. Gastroenterol. Hepatol.* **2012**, *24*, 1430–1437. [CrossRef] [PubMed]
68. Vortmeyer, A.O.; Lubensky, I.A.; Merino, M.J.; Wang, C.Y.; Pham, T.; Furth, E.E.; Zhuang, Z. Concordance of genetic alterations in poorly differentiated colorectal neuroendocrine carcinomas and associated adenocarcinomas. *J. Natl. Cancer Inst.* **1997**, *89*, 1448–1453. [CrossRef]
69. Tang, L.H.; Basturk, O.; Sue, J.J.; Klimstra, D.S. A practical approach to the classification of WHO grade 3 (G3) well differentiated neuroendocrine tumor (WD-NET) and poorly differentiated neuroendocrine carcinoma (PD-NEC) of the pancreas. *Am. J. Surg. Pathol.* **2016**, *40*, 1192–1202. [CrossRef]
70. Mafficini, A.; Scarpa, A. genetics and epigenetics of gastroenteropancreatic neuroendocrine neoplasms. *Endocr. Rev.* **2019**, *40*, 506–536. [CrossRef]

71. Ohmoto, A.; Rokutan, H.; Yachida, S. Pancreatic neuroendocrine neoplasms: Basic biology, current treatment strategies and prospects for the future. *Int. J. Mol. Sci.* **2017**, *18*, 143. [CrossRef] [PubMed]
72. Lamberti, G.; Brighi, N.; Maggio, I.; Manuzzi, L.; Peterle, C.; Ambrosini, V.; Ricci, C.; Casadei, R.; Campana, D. The role of mTOR in neuroendocrine tumors: future cornerstone of a winning strategy? *Int. J. Mol. Sci.* **2018**, *19*, 747. [CrossRef] [PubMed]
73. Lim, J.S.; Ibaseta, A.; Fischer, M.M.; Cancilla, B.; O'Young, G.; Cristea, S.; Luca, V.C.; Yang, D.; Jahchan, N.S.; Hamard, C.; et al. Intratumoural heterogeneity generated by Notch signalling promotes small-cell lung cancer. *Nature* **2017**, *545*, 360–364. [CrossRef] [PubMed]
74. Boora, G.K.; Kanwar, R.; Kulkarni, A.A.; Pleticha, J.; Ames, M.; Schroth, G.; Beutler, A.S.; Banck, M.S.; Gilbert, J.A. Exome-level comparison of primary well-differentiated neuroendocrine tumors and their cell lines. *Cancer Genet.* **2015**, *208*, 374–381. [CrossRef] [PubMed]
75. Palmer, W.H.; Jia, D.; Deng, W.M. Cis-interactions between Notch and its ligands block ligand-independent Notch activity. *eLife* **2014**, *3*. [CrossRef] [PubMed]
76. Wöltje, K.; Jabs, M.; Fischer, A. Serum induces transcription of Hey1 and Hey2 genes by Alk1 but not Notch signaling in endothelial cells. *PLoS ONE* **2015**, *10*, e0120547. [CrossRef] [PubMed]
77. Brzozowa-Zasada, M.; Piecuch, A.; Michalski, M.; Segiet, O.; Kurek, J.; Harabin-Słowińska, M.; Wojnicz, R. Notch and its oncogenic activity in human malignancies. *Eur. Surg.* **2017**, *49*, 199–209. [CrossRef] [PubMed]
78. Zou, B.; Zhou, X.L.; Lai, S.Q.; Liu, J.C. Notch signaling and non-small cell lung cancer. *Oncol. Lett.* **2018**, *15*, 3415–3421. [CrossRef] [PubMed]
79. Fukusumi, T.; Califano, J. The NOTCH pathway in head and neck squamous cell carcinoma. *J. Dent. Res.* **2018**, *97*, 645–653. [CrossRef] [PubMed]
80. Furuta, M.; Kikuchi, H.; Shoji, T.; Takashima, Y.; Kikuchi, E.; Kikuchi, J.; Kinoshita, I.; Dosaka-Akita, H.; Sakakibara-Konishi, J. DLL3 regulates the migration and invasion of small cell lung cancer by modulating Snail. *Cancer Sci.* **2019**, *110*, 1599–1608. [CrossRef] [PubMed]
81. Jaskula-Sztul, R.; Eide, J.; Tesfazghi, S.; Dammalapati, A.; Harrison, A.D.; Yu, X.M.; Scheinebeck, C.; Winston-McPherson, G.; Kupcho, K.R.; Robers, M.B.; et al. Tumor-suppressor role of Notch3 in medullary thyroid carcinoma revealed by genetic and pharmacological induction. *Mol. Cancer Ther.* **2015**, *14*, 499–512. [CrossRef] [PubMed]
82. Lobry, C.; Oh, P.; Mansour, M.R.; Look, A.T.; Aifantis, I. Notch signaling: Switching an oncogene to a tumor suppressor. *Blood* **2014**, *123*, 2451–2459. [CrossRef] [PubMed]
83. Crabtree, J.S.; Singleton, C.S.; Miele, L. Notch Signaling in neuroendocrine tumors. *Front. Oncol.* **2016**, *6*, 345. [CrossRef] [PubMed]
84. Harada, K.; Sato, Y.; Ikeda, H.; Hsü, M.; Igarashi, S.; Nakanuma, Y. Notch1-Hes1 signalling axis in the tumourigenesis of biliary neuroendocrine tumours. *J. Clin. Pathol.* **2013**, *66*, 386–391. [CrossRef] [PubMed]
85. Aster, J.C.; Pear, W.S.; Blacklow, S.C. The varied roles of notch in cancer. *Annu. Rev. Pathol.* **2017**, *12*, 245–275. [CrossRef]
86. Robinson, D.R.; Kalyana-Sundaram, S.; Wu, Y.M.; Shankar, S.; Cao, X.; Ateeq, B.; Asangani, I.A.; Iyer, M.; Maher, C.A.; Grasso, C.S.; et al. Functionally recurrent rearrangements of the mast kinase and notch gene families in breast cancer. *Nat. Med.* **2011**, *17*, 1646–1651. [CrossRef]
87. Stoeck, A.; Lejnine, S.; Truong, A.; Pan, L.; Wang, H.; Zang, C.; Yuan, J.; Ware, C.; MacLean, J.; Garrett-Engele, P.W.; et al. Discovery of biomarkers predictive of GSI response in triple negative breast cancer and adenoid cystic carcinoma. *Cancer Discov.* **2014**, *4*, 1154–1167. [CrossRef]
88. Parr, C.; Watkins, G.; Jiang, W.G. The possible correlation of Notch-1 and Notch-2 with clinical outcome and tumour clinicopathological parameters in human breast cancer. *Int. J. Mol. Med.* **2004**, *14*, 779–786. [CrossRef]
89. Wang, K.; Zhang, Q.; Li, D.; Ching, K.; Zhang, C.; Zheng, X.; Ozeck, M.; Shi, S.; Li, X.; Wang, H.; et al. PEST domain mutations in Notch receptors comprise an oncogenic driver segment in triple-negative breast cancer sensitive to a-secretase inhibitor. *Clin. Cancer Res.* **2015**, *21*, 1487–1496. [CrossRef]
90. Westhoff, B.; Colaluca, I.N.; D'Ario, G.; Donzelli, M.; Tosoni, D.; Volorio, S.; Pelosi, G.; Spaggiari, L.; Mazzarol, G.; Viale, G.; et al. Alterations of the Notch pathway in lung cancer. *Proc. Natl. Acad. Sci. USA* **2009**, *106*, 22293–22298. [CrossRef]

91. Zhu, J.; Wang, J.; Shi, Z.; Franklin, J.L.; Deane, N.G.; Coffey, R.J.; Beauchamp, R.D.; Zhang, B. Deciphering genomic alterations in colorectal cancer through transcriptional subtype-based network analysis. *PLoS ONE* **2013**, *8*, e79282. [CrossRef] [PubMed]
92. Mao, L. NOTCH Mutations: Multiple faces in human malignancies. *Cancer Prev. Res.* **2015**, *8*, 259–261. [CrossRef] [PubMed]
93. Xing, D.; Zheng, G.; Schoolmeester, J.K.; Li, Z.; Pallavajjala, A.; Haley, L.; Conner, M.G.; Vang, R.; Hung, C.F.; Wu, T.C.; et al. Next-generation sequencing reveals recurrent somatic mutations in small cell neuroendocrine carcinoma of the uterine cervix. *Am. J. Surg. Pathol.* **2018**, *42*, 750–760. [CrossRef] [PubMed]
94. Derks, J.L.; Leblay, N.; Lantuejoul, S.; Dingemans, A.M.C.; Speel, E.J.M.; Fernandez-Cuesta, L.; Speel, E. New insights into the molecular characteristics of pulmonary carcinoids and large cell neuroendocrine carcinomas, and the impact on their clinical management. *J. Thorac. Oncol.* **2018**, *13*, 752–766. [CrossRef] [PubMed]
95. Fernandez-Cuesta, L.; Peifer, M.; Lu, X.; Sun, R.; Ozretić, L.; Seidal, D.; Zander, T.; Leenders, F.; George, J.; Müller, C.; et al. Frequent mutations in chromatin-remodelling genes in pulmonary carcinoids. *Nat. Commun.* **2014**, *5*, 3518. [CrossRef] [PubMed]
96. Cives, M.; Simone, V.; Rizzo, F.M.; Silvestris, F. NETs: Organ-related epigenetic derangements and potential clinical applications. *Oncotarget* **2016**, *7*, 57414–57429. [CrossRef] [PubMed]
97. Kim, J.T.; Li, J.; Jang, E.R.; Gulhati, P.; Rychahou, P.G.; Napier, D.L.; Wang, C.; Weiss, H.L.; Lee, E.Y.; Anthony, L.; et al. Deregulation of Wnt/β-catenin signaling through genetic or epigenetic alterations in human neuroendocrine tumors. *Carcinogenesis* **2013**, *34*, 953–961. [CrossRef]
98. Graves, C.A.; Jones, A.; Reynolds, J.; Stuart, J.; Pirisi, L.; Botrous, P.; Wells, J. Neuroendocrine Merkel cell carcinoma is associated with mutations in key DNA repair, epigenetic and apoptosis pathways: A case-based study using targeted massively parallel sequencing. *Neuroendocrinology* **2015**, *101*, 112–119. [CrossRef]
99. Augert, A.; Eastwood, E.; Ibrahim, A.H.; Wu, N.; Grunblatt, E.; Basom, R.; Liggitt, D.; Eaton, K.D.; Martins, R.; Poirier, J.T.; et al. Targeting NOTCH activation in small cell lung cancer through LSD1 inhibition. *Sci. Signal* **2019**, *12*. [CrossRef] [PubMed]
100. Abraham, K.J.; Zhang, X.; Vidal, R.; Paré, G.C.; Feilotter, H.E.; Tron, V.A. Roles for miR-375 in neuroendocrine differentiation and tumor suppression via Notch pathway suppression in Merkel cell carcinoma. *Am. J. Pathol.* **2016**, *186*, 1025–1035. [CrossRef]
101. Arvidsson, Y.; Rehammar, A.; Bergström, A.; Andersson, E.; Altiparmak, G.; Swärd, C.; Wängberg, B.; Kristiansson, E.; Nilsson, O. miRNA profiling of small intestinal neuroendocrine tumors defines novel molecular subtypes and identifies miR-375 as a biomarker of patient survival. *Mod. Pathol.* **2018**, *31*, 1302–1317. [CrossRef] [PubMed]
102. Chiappinelli, K.B.; Zahnow, C.A.; Ahuja, N.; Baylin, S.B. Combining epigenetic and immunotherapy to combat cancer. *Cancer Res.* **2016**, *76*, 1683–1689. [CrossRef] [PubMed]
103. Meder, L.; König, K.; Ozretić, L.; Schultheis, A.M.; Ueckeroth, F.; Ade, C.P.; Albus, K.; Boehm, D.; Rommerscheidt-Fuss, U.; Florin, A.; et al. NOTCH, ASCL1, p53 and RB alterations define an alternative pathway driving neuroendocrine and small cell lung carcinomas. *Int. J. Cancer* **2016**, *38*, 927–938. [CrossRef] [PubMed]
104. Saunders, L.R.; Bankovich, A.J.; Anderson, W.C.; Aujay, M.A.; Bheddah, S.; Black, K.; Desai, R.; Escarpe, P.A.; Hampl, J.; Laysang, A.; et al. A DLL3-targeted antibody-drug conjugate eradicates high-grade pulmonary neuroendocrine tumor-initiating cells in vivo. *Sci. Transl. Med.* **2015**, *7*. [CrossRef] [PubMed]
105. Wang, H.; Chen, Y.; Fernandez-Del Castillo, C.; Yilmaz, O.; Deshpande, V. Heterogeneity in signaling pathways of gastroenteropancreatic neuroendocrine tumors: A critical look at notch signaling pathway. *Mod. Pathol.* **2013**, *26*, 139–147. [CrossRef] [PubMed]
106. Hanlon, L.; Avila, J.L.; Demarest, R.M.; Troutman, S.; Allen, M.; Ratti, F.; Rustgi, A.K.; Stanger, B.Z.; Radtke, F.; Adsay, V.; et al. Notch1 functions as a tumor suppressor in a model of K-ras-induced pancreatic ductal adenocarcinoma. *Cancer Res.* **2010**, *70*, 4280–4286. [CrossRef] [PubMed]
107. Miyamoto, Y.; Maitra, A.; Ghosh, B.; Zechner, U.; Argani, P.; Iacobuzio-Donahue, C.A.; Sriuranpong, V.; Iso, T.; Meszoely, I.M.; Wolfe, M.S.; et al. Notch mediates TGF alpha-induced changes in epithelial differentiation during pancreatic tumorigenesis. *Cancer Cell* **2003**, *3*, 565–576. [CrossRef]
108. Maggi, E.C.; Trillo-Tinoco, J.; Struckhoff, A.P.; Vijayaraghavan, J.; Del Valle, L.; Crabtree, J.S. Retinoblastoma-binding protein 2 (RBP2) is frequently expressed in neuroendocrine tumors and promotes the neoplastic phenotype. *Oncogenesis* **2016**, *5*, e257. [CrossRef]

109. Sippel, R.S.; Carpenter, J.E.; Kunnimalaiyaan, M.; Chen, H. The role of human achaete-scute homolog-1 in medullary thyroid cancer cells. *Surgery* **2003**, *134*, 866–871. [CrossRef]
110. Kunnimalaiyaan, M.; Vaccaro, A.M.; Ndiaye, M.A.; Chen, H. Overexpression of the NOTCH1 intracellular domain inhibits cell proliferation and alters the neuroendocrine phenotype of medullary thyroid cancer cells. *J. Biol. Chem.* **2006**, *281*, 39819–39830. [CrossRef]
111. Somnay, Y.R.; Yu, X.M.; Lloyd, R.V.; Leverson, G.; Aburjania, Z.; Jang, S.; Jaskula-Sztul, R.; Chen, H. Notch3 expression correlates with thyroid cancer differentiation, induces apoptosis, and predicts disease prognosis. *Cancer* **2017**, *123*, 769–782. [CrossRef] [PubMed]
112. Danza, G.; Di Serio, C.; Rosati, F.; Lonetto, G.; Sturli, N.; Kacer, D.; Pennella, A.; Ventimiglia, G.; Barucci, R.; Piscazzi, A.; et al. Notch signaling modulates hypoxia-induced neuroendocrine differentiation of human prostate cancer cells. *Mol. Cancer Res.* **2012**, *10*, 230–238. [CrossRef] [PubMed]
113. Puca, L.; Gavyert, K.; Sailer, V.; Conteduca, V.; Dardenne, E.; Sigouros, M.; Isse, K.; Kearney, M.; Vosoughi, A.; Fernandez, L.; et al. Delta-like protein 3 expression and therapeutic targeting in neuroendocrine prostate cancer. *Sci. Transl. Med.* **2019**, *11*. [CrossRef] [PubMed]
114. Jang, S.; Jin, H.; Roy, M.; Ma, A.L.; Gong, S.; Jaskula-Sztul, R.; Chen, H. Antineoplastic effects of histone deacetylase inhibitors in neuroendocrine cancer cells are mediated through transcriptional regulation of Notch1 by activator protein. *Cancer Med.* **2017**, *6*, 2142–2452. [CrossRef] [PubMed]
115. Mohammed, T.A.; Holen, K.D.; Jaskula-Sztul, R.; Mulkerin, D.; Lubner, S.J.; Schelman, W.R.; Eickhoff, J.; Chen, H.; LoConte, N.K. A Pilot Phase II Study of valproic acid for treatment of low-grade neuroendocrine carcinoma. *Oncologist* **2011**, *16*, 835–843. [CrossRef] [PubMed]
116. Sun, L.; Qian, Q.; Sun, G.; Mackey, L.V.; Fuselier, J.A.; Coy, D.H.; Yu, C.Y. Valproic acid induces NET cell growth arrest and enhances tumor suppression of the receptor-targeted peptide-drug conjugate via activating somatostatin receptor type II. *J. Drug Target.* **2016**, *24*, 169–177. [CrossRef] [PubMed]
117. Li, K.; Li, Y.; Wu, W.; Gordon, W.R.; Chang, D.W.; Lu, M.; Scoggin, S.; Fu, T.; Vien, L.; Histen, G.; et al. Modulation of Notch signaling by antibodies specific for the extracellular negative regulatory region of NOTCH3. *J. Biol. Chem.* **2008**, *283*, 8046–8054. [CrossRef] [PubMed]
118. Yen, W.C.; Fischer, M.M.; Axelrod, F.; Bond, C.; Cain, J.; Cancilla, B.; Henner, W.R.; Meisner, R.; Sato, A.; Shah, J.; et al. Targeting Notch signaling with a Notch2/Notch3 antagonist (Tarextumab) inhibits tumor growth and decreases tumor-initiating cell frequency. *Clin. Cancer Res.* **2015**, *21*, 2084–2095. [CrossRef] [PubMed]
119. Tolcher, A.W.; Messersmith, W.A.; Mikulski, S.M.; Papadopoulos, K.P.; Kwak, E.L.; Gibbon, D.G.; Patnaik, A.; Falchook, G.S.; Dasari, A.; Shapiro, G.I.; et al. Phase I study of RO4929097, a gamma secretase inhibitor of notch signaling, in patients with refractory metastatic or locally advanced solid tumors. *J. Clin. Oncol.* **2012**, *30*, 2348–2353. [CrossRef] [PubMed]
120. Carbone, D.P.; Morgenszstern, D.; Le Moulec, S.; Santana-Davila, R.; Ready, N.; Hann, C.L.; Glisson, B.S.; Dowlati, A.; Rudin, C.M.; Lally, S.; et al. Efficacy and safety of rovalpituzumab tesirine (Rova-TTM) in patients with DLL3-expressing, ≥3rd line small cell lung cancer: Results from the phase 2 TRINITY study. *J. Clin. Oncol.* **2018**, *36* (Suppl. S15), 8507. [CrossRef]
121. Phase 3 Trial of Rova-T as Second-Line Therapy for Advanced Small-Cell Lung Cancer (Tahoe Study) Halted. 2018. Available online: https://bit.ly/2KZcyVl (accessed on 6 December 2018).
122. Rudin, C.M.; Pietanza, M.C.; Bauer, T.M.; Ready, N.; Morgenszstern, D.; Glisson, B.S.; Byers, L.A.; Johnson, M.L.; Burris, H.A., III; Robert, F.; et al. Rovalpituzumab tesirine, a DLL3-targeted antibody-drug conjugate, in recurrent small-cell lung cancer: A first-in-human, first-in-class, open-label, phase 1 study. *Lancet Oncol.* **2017**, *18*, 42–51. [CrossRef]
123. Puca, L.; Sailor, V.; Gavyert, K.; Dardenne, E.; Isse, K.; Sigouros, M.; Nanus, D.M.; Tagawa, S.T.; Mosquera, J.M.; Saunders, L.; et al. Abstract 1947: Rovalpituzumab tesirine as a therapeutic agent for neuroendocrine prostate cancer. *Exp. Mol. Ther.* **2018**, *78*, 1947.
124. Chiu, M.L.; Gilliland, G.L. Engineering antibody therapeutics. *Curr. Opin. Struct. Biol.* **2016**, *38*, 163–173. [CrossRef] [PubMed]

125. Paramonov, V.M.; Desai, D.; Mamaeva, V.; Rosenholm, J.; Rivero-Müller, A.; Sahlgren, C. Mesoporous silica nanoparticles for somatostatin targeted Notch activation in animal model of pancreatic neuroendocrine cancer. *Endocr. Abstr.* **2016**, *40*. [CrossRef]
126. Fu, W.; Lei, C.; Yu, Y.; Liu, S.; Li, T.; Lin, F.; Fan, X.; Shen, Y.; Ding, M.; Tang, Y.; et al. EGFR/Notch antagonists enhance the response to inhibitors of the PI3K-Akt pathway by decreasing tumor-initiating cell frequency. *Clin. Cancer Res.* **2019**, *25*, 2835–2847. [CrossRef] [PubMed]

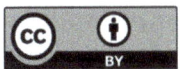

© 2019 by the authors. Licensee MDPI, Basel, Switzerland. This article is an open access article distributed under the terms and conditions of the Creative Commons Attribution (CC BY) license (http://creativecommons.org/licenses/by/4.0/).

MDPI
St. Alban-Anlage 66
4052 Basel
Switzerland
Tel. +41 61 683 77 34
Fax +41 61 302 89 18
www.mdpi.com

Journal of Clinical Medicine Editorial Office
E-mail: jcm@mdpi.com
www.mdpi.com/journal/jcm

www.ingramcontent.com/pod-product-compliance
Lightning Source LLC
LaVergne TN
LVHW070604100526
838202LV00012B/555